Communication for Doctors

How to improve patient care and minimize legal risks

Radcliffe Publishing Ltd
18 Marcham Road
Abingdon
Oxon OX14 1AA
United Kingdom

www.radcliffe-oxford.com
Electronic catalog and online worldwide ordering facility.

British Library Cataloging in Publication Data

A catalog record for this book is available from the British Library.

ISBN 1 85775 895 1

Typeset by Anne Joshua & Associates, Oxford, UK
Printed and bound by TJ International Ltd, Padstow, Cornwall, UK

Contents

Foreword

Physicians generally are blessed with, and educated to have, many skills but, unfortunately, effective communications skills and the ability to write clearly often seem to be missing from their list of abilities. Editor David Woods addresses these absent or weakly developed skills with humor and the insight of a gifted writer in this collection of physician communication advice. There is something for everyone here and no reader of this wonderful, witty, and thought provoking collection will fail to gain insight into how to improve his or her communication skills with patients and others. David Woods and his co-contributors present us with a wonderful menu of delicacies, a sumptuous communication feast guaranteed to satisfy the appetite of every physician who wishes to become a better communicator. The contributors' distinctive writing styles only add to this collection's diverse flavors. It is a book to be dipped into and savored piece by piece, and need not be read from cover-to-cover in one sitting.

Despite the personal nature of their professional calling, and a better than average educational background, physicians as a group frequently are charged with serious deficiencies in their writing and communication skills and abilities. Physicians have been accused of filling their written material with confused thought and ambiguity, ungrammatical and pretentious written constructions, medical jargon, and a too frequent tendency to pontification. Other cited physician writing shortcomings are a tendency to write to impress rather than to inform readers, and a fondness for technical terms to the exclusion of simpler words which would help reader understanding. Physicians who wish to develop good writing and communicating skills must learn to avoid ambiguity, wordiness, imprecision, vagueness, disorganization, pomposity, and writing clutter that ensures that no noun or verb goes unmodified in the writing. The ability to write well is not a natural talent for most physicians, hence it takes a dedicated effort by those physicians who wish to become more effective writers.

The purpose of physician writing is to communicate information of importance to patients, colleagues, and other readers, and its intrinsic value lies in the message it conveys, the questions it raises, and the thinking behind the decisions it announces. In medical writing for whatever purpose, the message conveyed by the writing always must be dominant. Medical writing must satisfy the reader's need for information, not the physician writer's need for self-expression. Good physician writers understand that effective writing skills afford them a unique opportunity for learning and teaching, and for persuading others. They possess a sense of audience which directs them to write from a reader's point of view, and which enables them to keep the reader's needs for information foremost in mind. In the long view, better physician communication and enhanced patient compliance with treatment recommendations depend, in great part, on the realization by physicians that producing competent and clear prose is part of the solution.

Physician writers, because of an inherent responsibility to their readers to convey clear and accurate information, can fulfill this responsibility to readers best by using precise rather than vague, and concrete rather than abstract, words to gain clarity of expression and meaning. Clarity of writing usually follows clarity of thought, so physician writers must think carefully about what they want to write, then write it as simply and clearly as possible. In medical writing, as in medical practice, being 'almost right' can be dangerous. Absolute accuracy in what is put into the writing is essential to good patient care. Good physician writing reflects the physician's ability to think logically, and physicians who learn good writing skills combine clear thinking with common language so that all readers understand clearly the meaning of what has been written.

The content matter of medical communications concerns itself with critical issues such as the health and welfare of a patient. Regardless of specialty or professional calling, all physicians require a common foundation of knowledge, values, professional attitudes, and basic clinical skills, including the ability to communicate effectively with patients and other physicians. Obtaining information from patients, communicating information to patients, and sharing information with colleagues is inherent in the practice of medicine. The fundamental rule of good physician writing is that the information presented to readers in the writing must be so clear and complete that it cannot be either misinterpreted or misunderstood by the reader.

Language is the essential, and perhaps the only, medium by which information and ideas are transferred from one mind to another. The first requirement of language is that it needs to be understood. The second requirement of language is that the information or ideas transferred by the language from one person to another person should not be distorted in the transfer process by factors such as faulty grammar, imprecise terms, poor word choice, disorganized sentence structure, or a difficult to follow writing style. The precise and accurate transfer of information by whatever means selected is a goal all physicians should embrace, and strive constantly to achieve.

A very pleasant journey awaits you – so, read, enjoy, and learn.

John J Gartland MD
June 2004

Preface

Look wise, say nothing, and grunt. Speech was given to conceal thought.

So said the great clinician Sir William Osler in the early part of the last century. And even if that piece of advice was offered tongue in cheek, today's physicians would quickly face opprobrium – if not a lawsuit – if they followed it.

As a matter of fact, litigation in medicine often has more to do with breakdown in communication than with clinical malfeasance. As Levinson *et al.* point out in the *Journal of the American Medical Association* (**277** (7): 553): "Significant differences in communication behaviors of no-claims and claims physicians were identified in primary care physicians." General internists and family doctors who spend more time with patients were more likely, according to the article, to educate them, to elicit information and to listen to it, and were less likely to face litigation.

And Maguire and Pitkeathly noted in the *British Medical Journal* (**325**: 697–700) that "good doctors communicate effectively with patients – they identify patients' problems more accurately, and patients are more satisfied with the care they receive." Moreover, the authors noted, doctors with good communication skills also have greater job satisfaction and less work stress.

It was with these kinds of thoughts in mind that I wrote *Paging Doctors*, a book largely about communication issues in healthcare – speaking, writing, reading, listening – and about the use, and misuse, of language in medicine. Out of that book came a newsletter, *Medical Practice Communicator*, which for eight years was sponsored by an enlightened medical malpractice insurance company that made it available to its 25 000 insured physicians.

While most of the pieces collected here are from that newsletter, some, especially the interview with Norman Cousins and the article on medicine and the English language, had an earlier life in *Paging Doctors* . . . and an even prior iteration in the pages of the *Canadian Medical Association Journal*, for which I wrote some 200 articles, editorials, reviews and interviews.

The medical director of that company, Dr Robert Pendrak, was the visionary who saw that physicians who communicate effectively are less likely to be sued. Since this book, *Communication for Doctors*, contains many of the articles that appeared in *Medical Practice Communicator*, I should like also to acknowledge here the newsletter's vigilant and talented copy-editor and proofreader, Edith Schwager, author of *Medical English Usage and Abusage*, and its equally rigorous medical editor, Dr John Gartland, author of *Medical Writing and Communicating*. Further, I am most grateful for the contributions made by readability consultant, Mark Hochhauser; lawyers Joan Roediger and James Saxton; former scientific editor of the *Canadian Medical Association Journal*, Dr Peter Morgan; computer and information technology expert, Jonathan Coopersmith; Susan Keane Baker, author of *Managing Patient Expectations*; Albert Mehl, pediatrician; Julia Schopick, public relations consultant; and Peter Ubel, Director, Health Care Decisions

Program – all of whose work appears, with their permission, in the following pages. Further thanks are due to production editor, Norman Kline, for scanning and pulling together the 66 titles that make up *Communication for Doctors*, and to my wife, Shelly Wolf, for her project management skills, sage counsel, and unfailing support and encouragement.

All of us associated with *Medical Practice Communicator* felt that many of its articles were too valuable to the broader international community of medical practitioners to be allowed simply to float into the ether. That is why we have collected the best of them here – to help doctors become not only better communicators, but better doctors.

David Woods PhD
President, Healthcare Media International, Inc.
Philadelphia, PA
June 2004

About the editor

David Woods PhD is the founder (in 1993) and Chief Executive Officer of Healthcare Media International (HMI). HMI publishes periodicals on management, communication, risk management, and managed care, and provides consulting and editorial services in these areas, as well as on healthcare policy.

David holds a doctorate in healthcare policy from the University of Ulster's Faculty of Health and Social Sciences and Education, and is the author of three books on health policy, including *The Future of the Managed Care Industry and its International Implications*, published by the *Economist Intelligence Unit* in 1998.

A former editor of *Canadian Doctor* and *Canadian Family Physician*, he served for eight years as director of publications for the Canadian Medical Association, and as the first non-physician editor-in-chief of the *Canadian Medical Association Journal*, before moving to the United States in 1987. He is the author of several hundred articles, editorials, reviews, and interviews – more than 100 of which are cited in *Index Medicus*/MEDLINE (see under Woods, D).

David is a member of the British American Business Council, the Philadelphia County Medical Society's Editorial Board, and the Alliance Française. He also develops, and teaches, a graduate course in medical publishing at a Philadelphia-area university. He contributes regularly to the *British Medical Journal* and serves on the Board of Directors of the American Medical Publishers Association.

List of contributors

Susan Keane Baker
New Canaan, Connecticut
Author of *Managing Patient Expectations*

Jonathan Coopersmith
Information Technology Consultant
Philadelphia, Pennsylvania

John Gartland MD
Medical Editor
Thomas Jefferson University
Author of *Medical Writing and Communicating*

Mark Hochhauser PhD
Readability Consultant
Golden Valley, Minnesota

Albert Mehl MD
Pediatrician
Boulder, Colorado

Peter Morgan MD
Former Scientific Editor
Canadian Medical Association Journal
Lanark, Ontario, Canada

Robert Pendrak MD
Director of Risk Management
Inservco Insurance Services
Harrisburg, Pennsylvania

Joan Roediger JD
Attorney
Obermayer Rebmann Maxwell and Hippel, LLP
Philadelphia, Pennsylvania

James Saxton JD
Attorney
Smith and Lee
Lancaster, Pennsylvania
Author of *Managed Care Success*

Julia E Schopick
Public Relations Consultant
Oak Park, Illinois

Peter E Ubel MD
Director, Health Care Decisions Program
University of Michigan
Ann Arbor, Michigan

National Council on Patient Information and Education
Bethesda, Maryland

Patients are a virtue

What do patients think of doctors as communicators?

While patients tend to like their own doctors, most have a poor image of doctors as a group. The public's opinion that doctors are not good communicators, at least as far as the public's own health needs are concerned, adds to this poor image. Despite the personal nature of medical care and the lengthy educational process required, often patients perceive physicians as having serious deficiencies in their communication and interpersonal skills.

All too often, doctors seem to lack the ability to write clearly, speak effectively in professional settings, or use language that patients and others can readily understand. Poor communication with patients and others can cause medical information to be misinterpreted or misunderstood, and this can result in inappropriate or ineffective patient care and even an increase in malpractice suits. Many patients think doctors are arrogant, and do not believe they do an effective job in either communicating information to them about their illness or expressing concern about their welfare as patients. If such views and opinions are widespread, it is not surprising that some medical care outcomes, as viewed by patients, are less than optimal. Evidence exists that medical care, despite its professional and technical advances, may not be meeting the needs of patients, and the reason is believed to be lack of effective doctor–patient communication.

Good communication with patients is a principal cornerstone of effective and satisfying medical care. Many problems between doctors and patients have their origin in the doctor's lack of balance between an emphasis on curing and an emphasis on caring. More than ever before, doctors now must recognize and appreciate how large a part their interpersonal and communication skills play in the delivery of good medical care. True compassion for the health problems of patients is really a product of sensitive and aware communication.

Patients' satisfaction with a medical experience is an important determinant of their cooperation with recommended treatment plans, and that depends more on how the doctor's communication skills are perceived than on anything else. In turn, patient satisfaction with a medical experience relates more to the doctor's communication skills than to the perceived quality of the medical care, the patient's waiting time, or even the cost of the care. Many patients will rate their medical experience as unsatisfactory if the doctor gives them little information. Patients frequently complain that when doctors do offer explanations to them, these explanations are difficult to understand because the doctor uses obscure language and medical jargon. How well or how poorly doctors communicate with patients has a direct bearing on the accuracy of their diagnoses, and the compliance, satisfaction with and response to treatment of their patients.

John Gartland MD

Making patients your partners

The concept of pleasing patients, being customer-oriented, and involving patients in their own care (which will also drive customer satisfaction) has been underrated. Although much has been written about this concept and it is the subject of many lectures, it has not caught enough attention at the operational level.

Making patients partners is more than a cliché. It means looking at how you can achieve a greater level of patient involvement and understanding of their care. It takes looking at what information they need and how best to promote it. It could be as simple as looking at patient information pamphlets or postoperative instructions with an eye toward whether they are understandable to someone with an eighth-grade education. It may be something as simple as inviting a small cross-section of your patients into your office over a lunch hour to review your patient education material and to tell you whether it's helpful or unclear. What questions have been left unanswered? What further information would patients need so that they can truly understand the information you are trying to convey?

It could be more sophisticated, such as creating a patient journal with a care map that a patient needs to follow in handling a particular disease, such as diabetes or urinary incontinence, and working with patients to show them and their families how they can be active participants.

Studies have shown that patients who are more involved and more connected with their care comply more and fare better. They are more satisfied and rate their doctors higher in satisfaction surveys. There is a direct positive correlation between how involved patients are in their care and your risk of a professional liability lawsuit.

There are just too many reasons to be more creative and take more time and resources to determine how to make this important topic more operational in your practice.

You can start now by looking at your patient satisfaction results. If you have not conducted a survey, do so within the next six months. If a full patient satisfaction survey seems too cumbersome, have a focus group survey and review your educational materials. You can then make revisions. Provide some training to the staff and physicians.

If you have not provided an educational opportunity for your staff in the last 12 months on communication skill or patient satisfaction, you have failed to provide them with the tools needed. Choose two or three key aspects of customer satisfaction to work on this year.

David Woods

Thirty ways to make your practice more "patient-friendly"

There are many quick and easy ways to make your practice more "patient-friendly." As you read this list, note the five ideas that make the most sense for you – and put them to use today!

1 People like people who speak first. Don't wait for your patients to introduce themselves – take the initiative.
2 For first-time patients, have a preliminary meeting before beginning any testing or treatment.
3 Try to speak to your patient on the same physical level. In hospitals, two minutes sitting by the bed is worth more to the patient than ten minutes standing in the doorway.
4 Use words that are familiar and comfortable for the patient. If your patient uses "terrific," let your statement be "I think you are doing a terrific job with your diet – you must be proud of yourself."
5 Don't assume that your patient understands even the most basic medical terminology. Yes, people watch medical-themed soap operas, but they don't watch television with a medical dictionary in hand. Keep this in mind even when caring for patients employed in the health professions. One office nurse, new to a pediatric practice, thought that the bilirubin results were for a patient called Billy Rubin.
6 Keep notes on your patients' individual preferences – early morning appointments, for example. Customers value relationships where their individual preferences are acknowledged.
7 Address all adult patients by their last names, unless they ask you to use their first names. This is particularly pertinent to older patients.
8 Give written information for even the simplest advice. This is a major patient satisfier – and it means fewer questions later.
9 Everyone in the practice should review the appointment schedule at the beginning of the day. A patient can then be greeted by name.
10 Instead of asking "Do you have any questions?" try "What questions can I answer for you?"
11 Try to mirror the patient's pace and tone of voice, except when the patient is angry or afraid.
12 Patients see and feel the practice's atmosphere. So make positive statements and recognition of client service part of your organizational culture. Tom Peters, author and lecturer on excellence in business, recommends that dozens of opportunities be provided to inform staff about customer service.

13 Remember the power of appropriate touch. Offering to hold a patient's hand or patting a patient's arm during an uncomfortable procedure is long remembered by patients.

14 Recognize significant events in your patient's life. If you see a news article or wedding announcement, for example, clip it out and send it with a quick note.

15 Be clear about what will happen next. "Your test results will be back in a week" leaves your patient wondering "Will the doctor call me, or am I supposed to call her?" Be specific about what you will do after the visit, and what your patient will do.

16 Consider presurgical and follow-up telephone calls. The surgeon who calls the night before surgery and says, "I've been thinking about you today and wonder if you have any questions about tomorrow," is a special person.

17 Everyone likes to be right. See if you can use the phrase "You're right" once during each patient visit. It can be as simple as "You're right, Mrs Jones, it is a beautiful day."

18 Smile! Make your patients feel that you are happy to see them. Greet them with the same smile you would use to greet a guest to your home.

19 Respond as quickly as possible to patient requests. A quick response differentiates you from all other physicians providing the same service, and it will make your patient feel important.

20 Let patients see that you are taking precautions for their benefit. Instead of walking into the examination room wearing gloves, let them see you putting gloves on.

21 To achieve a trusting relationship, your patient has to know that confidentiality will be respected by you and your staff. Make confidentiality an obsession and find ways to communicate your values to your patients.

22 Would you like to have you as a healthcare provider? Why or why not? Start doing more of the "why" things and fewer "why nots."

23 Whenever possible, let telephone callers hang up first.

24 Patients want to feel that their healthcare providers spend enough time with them. You can create the impression that a meaningful amount of time was spent by giving undivided attention to your patient during the first 60 seconds of your encounter. It's not as easy as it sounds.

25 Just say yes.

26 Think about how you felt on your first day of practice and let your patients see your enthusiasm. People love people who love what they do.

27 Think about what you can do for your patient and let your patient know. "We'll use this examining room today – it's warmer than the others."

28 Consider the group you most like to do business with – why? Can you duplicate the experience?

29 Before beginning a procedure with a patient, ask, "Is there anything I can do to make you more comfortable before we begin?"

30 Be a star with your patients. Going the extra mile does not necessarily mean a lot of extra effort. It just requires caring and thinking about your patients' needs.

Susan Keane Baker

Eight easy ways to make the medicine go down

Numerous studies during the past decade have shown that doctors who take the time to talk to their patients about their medicines are likely to have more compliant patients. Researchers have also found that anywhere from 20% to 33% of all patients get no oral instructions about their prescriptions from pharmacists. Still other studies have concluded that health professionals over-estimate how well their patients comply with drug regimens by as much as 50%. Here are eight ways to make the medicine go down:

1   *Target your intervention.* Spend your time and energy on the patients least likely to be able to comply on their own – particularly the elderly who live alone and patients who have to take many drugs or have complex regimens to follow. Consider paying close attention to patients for whom non-compliance might mean a trip to the emergency room or a stay in hospital.
2   *Delegate.* Use your office staff. Make arrangements with case workers or with local pharmacists to whom you can refer patients for special education or intervention.
3   *Take advantage of technology.* There are all sorts of low- and high-tech compliance tools on the market, including bottle caps that count, electronic pill boxes that beep, and unit-dose blister packs. There are private companies that use computers and case managers to promote compliance with particular patients. Insurance companies are sometimes willing to pay for such services if a cost-effectiveness argument can be made.
4   *Give patients more information.* Studies have found that giving patients information is a necessary, if insufficient, intervention. There are, however, a few ways to improve the chances a patient will hear, understand, and accept a regimen. These include discussing the most important information first, repeating key points, having the patient restate key instructions, and asking nurses and pharmacists to repeat instructions. Combine oral and written explanations. Emphasize the theme that patients have the responsibility for self-care.
5   *Refer to support groups.* Some health centers and office practices have been able to improve compliance among the elderly by recruiting particular patients into support groups.
6   *Listen.* You are looking for clues to the underlying reasons for their non-compliance. Try to avoid making the act of writing the prescription the signal that the visit is about to end.
7   *Make it easy.* Prescribe twice-a-day medications whenever possible. Send appointment reminders. Increase the frequency of visits to take advantage of the "white coat" effect, which makes patients reluctant to lie to the doctor when asked if they have been taking their medicine as prescribed.

8   *Don't reinvent the wheel.* There are many organizations that have thoughts about this issue. Ask your drug company detailers, pharmacists, hospital case management staffs, and managed-care organizations what help they can offer patients who have difficulty complying with treatment plans.

National Council on Patient Information and Education

Answering questions patients don't ask

Almost all patients have questions they want to ask their doctors, but don't. Depending on the patient, there may be various reasons for this reticence. A patient may be confused or anxious, especially after being told of a serious condition. Or that patient may be intimidated and feel that whatever the physician says and decides to do should not be questioned. Older patients, and sometimes very young patients, may not be comfortable "questioning" the doctor.

Yet, ensuring that the patient is fully informed – and has no outstanding questions – is essential to the successful doctor–patient visit. Incorporating the following steps into your patient visits can help you make certain that the patient does not leave your office with unanswered questions:

- Never underestimate a patient's intelligence. Even relatively uneducated patients want to be fully informed about their health and any treatment prescribed. Be careful, however, to use a vocabulary appropriate to the patient's educational level, comprehension, and temperament.
- Explain what you are doing and why you are doing it. During a physical examination, for example, tell the patient, in a brief conversational manner, why you are listening to his or her chest; asking the patient in this way, you create an opportunity for the patient to ask questions and remember symptoms that were not elicited during the history taking.
- Discuss the diagnosis and the treatment regimen carefully and then encourage the patient to ask questions. If the patient fails to ask appropriate questions, ask questions yourself. Helpful ones include: Do you understand what [say] diabetes is now that we have discussed it? Do you have any questions about the treatment I am recommending for you? Are you sure you understand why I am recommending this particular medication?
- Empathize with the patient and try to elicit concerns and anxieties the patient may be reluctant to bring up. A patient who has just learned of a serious condition, for example, probably is feeling shock, anxiety, and concern about the prognosis. Leading comments such as "You are probably worried about what effect this will have on your life" will encourage the patient to express concerns and anxieties. Discussing these issues will help alleviate them and will also give you an opportunity to respond to questions that are uppermost in the patient's mind although he or she is hesitant to express them.
- Encourage the patient to telephone you if any questions arise after the patient has left your office.

Making sure that all of a patient's questions are answered, even those that often go unasked, may require special effort and understanding on your part, but the rewards are many.

The patient's stress and anxiety will be reduced because questions and concerns have been anticipated and answered. Compliance with prescribed treatment will improve because the patient understands the condition better and is aware of the reasons for and the benefits of treatment. The patient's level of trust in you and satisfaction with care will increase. As a result, your relationship with the patient will be strengthened, quality of care will be enhanced, and patient outcomes will be improved; the risk of malpractice suits will be reduced as well.

So the next time a patient has no more questions, don't believe it! Find out what the patient's unasked questions are and make sure they are answered before the patient leaves your office.

Can your patients read your writing?

How much education does it take to read (and understand) your writing? If you write at a graduate school level, fewer than 20% will understand your materials. If you write at a college level, about 20–40% will understand; if you write at a high-school level, about 75–90% will understand. To have over 90% of the public understand your materials, you should write at the level of a 12–13 year-old – or lower.

An "informed consent" form given to patients to test a new drug is written at a second- or third-year college reading level, making it understandable to less than 40% of the adult population. Evaluating your writing by using only a grade-level estimate is like trying to diagnose patients' conditions by simply taking their temperature. Detailed readability analyses can be done with the help of programs such as Grammatik 6.0, RightWriter 6.0, Correct Grammar, Readability Plus, PROSE, and FSText. Many of these are available as freeware or shareware through online services such as CompuServe and America Online.

That typical informed consent form was not only written at a second to third-year college reading level but it was "difficult, at the scientific level," "affirmative and mostly positive," and "very hard for the average reader." Over 40% of the sentences were written at a graduate school reading level. About 16% of the sentences were "complicated" (short sentences with long words) and 16% were "pompous" (long sentences with long words). One sentence was 57 words long. About 60% of the words were "small" (one syllable), while about 19% of the words were "big" (more than two syllables). On average, each sentence was about 25 words long.

The writing could be improved by using the active voice, writing shorter sentences, using fewer wordy phrases, and using more common words.

Some patients may cause problems. Perhaps you label them as "non-compliant" or "difficult," because they're not following your instructions or they don't seem motivated. Perhaps they cost you time and money because they frequently call you for information. Perhaps they just can't read or understand your writing.

Mark Hochhauser

How about a Hippocratic Oath for patients?

The medical profession has felt the need almost since its inception to be bound by a written code of duty, obligation, and behavior. But if one takes seriously the dictum of Herbert Spencer, the 19th century British philosopher who believed that no one can be perfectly moral until all are moral, then maybe the time has come to look at a code of ethics for patients.

Such a proposal, in light of today's easy-going and generally subjective approach to morality, might well be little more than idealistic velleity. Whether or not it gathers momentum will depend to a large extent on the patient. Of course one must first ask whether patients ever attempt to take advantage of doctors physically, emotionally, or financially. Well, we know that verbal doctor bashing is a fact of life, and that physical assaults on physicians by patients are on the increase; we know that more patients try to seduce their doctors than vice (if you'll forgive the expression) versa.

On the other hand, the patient's position *vis-à-vis* the doctor is usually distinctly subordinate – it is less easy to bargain with force and dignity when semi or totally unclad.

Nonetheless, patients do know that physicians are sworn to Hippocratic and other oaths; they also know that they are bound by no comparably documented proscriptions against licentiousness, litigation, and lying. The customer may not be physically or mentally right, but is generally assumed to be morally so.

A code of ethics for patients might serve to redress the imbalance, if not the inequity, that normally characterizes the purely medical aspects of the doctor–patient relationship.

It would start out with some reference to the physician's working hours, and how, even if the cough started at 3 a.m., treatment might be delayed until postdawn.

There could be something about giving a history that makes reasonable physiologic and linguistic sense.

It might go on to note that "an ethical patient . . . will take the medicine as directed." But also that common sense will take precedence over this particular ethic if the medicine in question causes the patient to turn blue – in which case prudence and self-protection will require telling the doctor.

It would remove all hospital privileges from patients who call women doctors "nurse." Those who recite Dorland's to any physician in a social setting, particularly dinner, would be required to listen to endless golfing stories.

What a contribution to the doctor–patient relationship.

David Woods

Hippocrates was right: treat people, not their disease

Ever since that first long night in the emergency department with my husband nearly 10 years ago, I have wanted to teach a course entitled "Life of the Patient; Life of the Family" to help doctors create more satisfying relationships with patients and patients' families and thus deliver the best possible care.

With each passing year, as my husband and I go through more treatments, hospitalizations and doctors' visits, I think about this course. I want to teach it because I continue to cross paths with many doctors who appear to have lost sight of Hippocrates' centuries-old observation that "what sort of person has a disease" is more important than "what sort of a disease a person has." In other words, although a doctor may know much about a person's illness, if he or she knows little about the person, little or no healing will take place.

What should doctors know to facilitate healing? More about their patients' home lives, problems resulting from their illnesses, how they feel about their illnesses – and this is just a beginning.

My dad, a general practitioner, learned about his patients through house calls and by careful listening. He believed that the more you knew about your patients, the better you could diagnose and successfully treat them. This was his secret: "I am like a detective and the patient and his family give me my clues. I want their opinions. Without listening, I can't help solve their problems."

Even though he was, in his words, "just a GP," my dad was often called in by specialists to help diagnose their "difficult" cases – most probably because of his listening skills.

When I talk with doctors today, some tell me they know they could do a better job if they had more time to understand their patients. But others don't see how understanding a patient's personal life is an important part of medical treatment.

Through the years, I have seen many situations where healing might have occurred, even though the doctor failed to understand or empathize with the patient. These doctors fell into the trap of "if you've seen one brain tumor or lung cancer patient, you've seen them all."

One dear friend first met his oncologist when his lung cancer had already metastasized to the liver. Without knowing anything about him, this doctor announced that my friend had only six months to live. He didn't know, or care, that my friend had a very satisfying home, work and spiritual life – and did not intend to die. This physician failed to understand that this patient was confronting his own illness and, in addition to prescribed treatments, was using his own means, both physical and mental, to help himself.

When my friend was still alive 18 months later, the doctor, seemingly frustrated by the fact that the patient hadn't abided by the prognosis, sent him to hospice!

Nevertheless, my friend is still alive now, six months later, two years after diagnosis – without hospice.

When I think of this oncologist, I recall how much my dad enjoyed the love, respect and devotion of his patients, and wish more doctors today could have similar experiences. I am convinced that getting involved in their patients' lives could give them some of that joy, and turn them into better healers.

It occurs to me that the fear of being sued may make today's doctors wary of involvement. But lack of involvement may actually be a large part of the reason they do get sued. One benefit of being more empathic with patients is that friends don't sue friends. I once asked my dad if he ever made mistakes. "You bet." I asked him if he'd ever been sued. "No, people don't sue the doctor who's by their bedside at 3 in the morning."

If I were to teach my course, what information would I include? Here are just a few of the lessons I would cover:

- Listen to your patients – and their families. It has been reported that doctors listen to patients for 18 seconds before interrupting. You will miss very important information this way.
- Find out what this illness has done to your patient and the family. Don't assume that understanding the disease process is enough. A patient with a brain tumor should not be defined by the size and grade of the tumor. Although that patient's tumor might look the same on a scan as another patient's, each person's experience will be different.
- Ask about your patient's home life. Just because your patient is always accompanied to office visits, don't assume all is well. Perhaps your patient is being brought to your office by a paid "keeper." This may not bode well for the patient's outcome.
- Ask how your patient's work life has been affected by this illness. Is this a long-standing illness? Is the patient able to work? If so, is he or she still earning the same salary? It is doubtful that this is the case, and if it isn't, your patient may be having financial troubles, which can add greatly to the stress.

These are just a few of the topics I would cover in my course. I hope that more and more doctors will begin to see the value of understanding their patients. It is this understanding and empathy that will bring joy back into physicians' lives and make them better healers.

Julia E Schopick

How non-verbal communication can give patients a sense of connectedness

Following a patient's quadruple bypass surgery, a friend met the surgeon in the hospital, who told him that things had gone well and predicted a rapid recovery. But the patient's wife was very upset. The surgeon, she said, never once looked at her while explaining her husband's condition but looked at the walls and ceiling during the explanation. He gave what he thought was a clear explanation but failed to include the recipient of the explanation in his communication. The non-verbal cues expressed by the surgeon's behavior suggested coldness and lack of interest to her – and triggered the anger.

Non-verbal cues expressed by physicians often mirror professional attitudes and have an effect on patient care. A critical component of good physician–patient relationships is the attentiveness displayed by physicians toward the information and non-verbal cues given by patients. Equally important are the non-verbal cues expressed by physicians who, more often than not, are unaware of expressing them and of their effect on patients. Non-verbal communication is used to communicate feelings, likings, attitudes, and preferences, and tends to reinforce or contradict feelings conveyed verbally. Good non-verbal communication by physicians is associated with patient satisfaction and understanding.

Few physicians consider the manner in which they communicate non-verbally with patients. But information given to patients and their families can be positively or negatively influenced by accompanying non-verbal cues expressed knowingly or unknowingly. The core of the physician–patient relationship is the ability of the participants to talk freely and openly with each other. Insightful and sensitive physicians have learned to interpret and respond to the nuances of both verbal and non-verbal communication exchanges between patients, their families, and themselves.

A physician's capacity for sending and receiving non-verbal messages by body posture, voice tone and inflection, facial expression, and eye contact is part of good communication. Listen to what patients have to say about themselves and make eye contact when speaking with them. Eyes focused in the direction of a conversation can reflect concern and encouragement, and reinforce a positive attitude. Looking directly at patients when speaking with them is interpreted by patients as a reflection of concern for their welfare and interest in the problem at hand. Physicians need to remember that, at best, medicine is not only a learned science but also a personal art. Good non-verbal communication skill reinforces communications and gives patients a sense of connectedness with their physicians.

John Gartland MD

Empowered patients may have something to teach us

Imagine this scenario: Your new patient is a 50-year-old man who was operated on for a cancerous brain tumor 10 years ago. There were several more surgeries to remedy complications, as well as the standard chemotherapy and radiation. He has been on a low dose of anti-seizure medication for several years, with some minor seizures in between. He is now in the hospital for "intractable seizures."

You want to put him on some stronger anti-seizure medications that his wife says he tolerated badly years ago. Three weeks have passed and it is crucial that these seizures be addressed.

His wife is frantic. And, hardly a stranger to medical research, she feels that her contribution and involvement in her husband's care have been at least partly responsible for his much-better-than-average recovery. She goes online, and also consults with friends and colleagues about this problem.

After several days, she approaches you with a possible solution: a newer medication that is not as "tried and true" as the ones you want to use, but is known to produce fewer cognitive side-effects.

Young Doctor No. 1 is miffed, and tells her that she is welcome to take her husband elsewhere if she doesn't trust the doctor's judgment. The wife, upset by this response, asks to see another physician – this time the head of the department.

Doctor No. 2 has a totally different approach. Realizing that this wife (by the way, I am the wife in this scenario) may have a new insight, he says, "This is an interesting possibility. I hadn't thought about trying that drug, but perhaps we should consider it. Let me think about it, and we'll talk."

How would you react – like Doctor No. 1 or Doctor No. 2?

If you reacted like Doctor No. 1, you would have lost an opportunity to work with a new but growing breed of patient and family member: those who are "empowered." You also would have opened yourself up to an adversarial position – which could, by the way, lead to a lawsuit later on.

With the advent of the Internet, coupled with publicity about the negative effects of many pharmaceutical drugs, and a growing interest in integrative (holistic, complementary or alternative) medicine, there are more and more patients and family members who are becoming empowered. Many doctors tell me that they are not sure how – or whether – to interact with these patients. But soon they may not have to decide, because increasing numbers of patients are, indeed, going online.

First, it is important to realize that many of your patients are probably already doing their own research, especially in relation to alternative therapies, including herbs and vitamins. Although they may not be telling you yet about the supplements they are taking, realize that they will probably start to be more open with you in the future.

One friend of mine decided that she would follow the radiation and chemo-therapy protocols her doctor recommended, but would supplement them with vitamins and herbs. Her doctor was open and supportive, and asked her about what she was taking, although he didn't do any research on his own.

My friend is doing extremely well four years post-treatment. She credits her success to a lot of prayer, as well as a combination of traditional and alternative treatments – and to a doctor who was supportive of her as a human being.

How should a doctor work with a patient who brings him (or her) information about treatments that are more holistic? I had an extremely positive experience recently – again with a new doctor. I brought him a hefty packet of information to read about a possible new holistic treatment for my husband. Although the doctor is an extremely busy man, he read the material and got back to me within five days, explaining the pluses (there were several) and the minuses (he didn't find any). He believed that it looked quite promising. This doctor and I have had many wonderful conversations and he tells me he finds our working together – and the results we are obtaining for my husband – exciting. So do I.

How should you work effectively with the empowered patient, given your time constraints and your possible lack of familiarity with some of the less traditional treatments?

- Show an interest. Ask which medications (including over-the-counter) your patients are taking; also ask about vitamins and herbs. To assume that there can be no harm in combining drugs and herbs can be a huge mistake. There can be interactions. On the other hand, many patients are finding that their traditional treatments are being enhanced through sound diet choices, as well as careful supplementation with vitamins, minerals and herbs. But there are right supplements and wrong supplements to take, depending on a patient's condition and on the drugs he or she is taking.
- Don't dismiss your patients' research. When a patient brings you articles (or sections from books), as well as downloaded selections from the Internet, don't automatically assume they lack merit; try to read them. If you are getting too many such requests on a regular basis, consider consulting with a researcher to assess the quality of the information your patients bring you, as well as to conduct research on medical topics of interest to you and your patients.
- Be happy that your patients are researching their treatments, because an involved patient most likely will do better in the long run. Teachers will tell you that the more involved students are in learning, the longer they will remember the material and the more meaningful it will be to them. The same goes for your patients.
- But, perhaps most important, working in a collaborative way with the empowered patient can actually be fun for both doctor and patient or family member, as well as lead to a much better result.

Julia E Schopick

How to communicate with patients who (think they) know more than you do

A generation ago, research results did not appear in the media before the latest medical journals were piled on the doctor's desk; pharmaceuticals were not advertised in the lay press; and disease-victim groups didn't exist. New findings aged quietly as they circulated through the medical network. Today, consumerism and advocacy have short-circuited the process, and the information pile of a concerned patient focused on a single chronic disorder may be higher and fresher than the physician's.

While physicians may welcome patients' efforts to become more knowledgeable, this can pose a challenge to the patient–doctor relationship if it is based on misinformation.

A focused review of current journals is an essential step for physicians who want to apply their understanding of the relevant basic science and ability to appraise the latest scientific evidence to the patients' concerns.

Suggested strategies for keeping up with (or ahead of) your patients include the following:

- Get an office assistant or family member to set up a newspaper clipping service targeted at breakthrough stories. Media sources do not always distinguish between pivotal studies that will change medical practice and preliminary findings, but they sometimes refer to the journal publishing the results. Recent articles appear promptly on the journals' websites, but likely not in MEDLINE in time for you to respond to a newspaper article.
- Read the contents pages of four weekly journals: *Lancet*, *New England Journal of Medicine*, *Journal of the American Medical Association*, and a journal of your choice. Check topics of interest and have an assistant photocopy the abstract for a topic file. Computer users can skim information from journal websites, but it takes as long as getting it from hard copy.
- If the patient's news sounds unfamiliar, but plausible, temporize: "You give me the source – I'll check it out and get back to you."
- If the patient refers to an untested or fringe theory, stake out the boundaries of your communication responsibility; admit that you don't take some systems and theories of healing seriously because they can't be tested scientifically.

Peter Morgan MD

How to deal with illiterate patients

The doctor explains. The patient nods.

The question is, does the patient really understand what the doctor is saying about the diagnosis and treatment plan? In very many cases the answer is no.

It's a question of medical literacy, or, more to the point, illiteracy. More than 40 million American adults are functionally illiterate, and an even greater number, 50 million, are only marginally literate. What happens when they become patients is that prescriptions are not taken correctly, treatment plans are ignored, and self-monitoring goes undone. All at a cost of increased suffering and many millions of dollars. In one hospital study, 42% of patients were unable to comprehend directions for taking medicine on an empty stomach, 26% could not understand information on an appointment slip, and 60% could not understand a standard consent form.

Health warnings and immunization notices are lost on someone who can't read them. The same applies to information about preparing for a test or procedure, or about what symptoms should prompt a visit to the doctor.

All this comes at a time when both medical advances and cost consciousness in the health system have raised expectations that patients will take a more active role in the monitoring and treatment of their illnesses.

Physicians can play a significant role in addressing this problem by being aware that many patients try to hide the fact that they can't read. Doctors should make instructions simple and clear, and communicate interactively. Show the patient a pill bottle and ask, "If this were your medicine, tell me, how would you take it?"

Literacy is a fundamental issue for the medical profession. The marvels of modern medicine don't amount to much for patients who can't master something as simple as taking the right pill at the right time.

David Woods

How to avoid alienating patients

Recently, my husband became seriously ill, requiring many visits to doctors in several specialties. I had the opportunity to view the medical profession not in my role as a public relations counsel to that profession, but as the wife of a patient.

Listen to your patients

My father, a general practitioner, often said he saw himself as a detective. The clues were provided by his patients and their families, so that together they could solve the puzzle and treat the disease. How unnerving, then, to find that many of the doctors we dealt with were simply not good listeners.

One oncologist we saw did not seem to be interested in listening to my husband or to me. When he or I spoke, she would write, walk around the room, or otherwise appear to be totally uninterested. I doubt that she gave it a second thought when we decided to seek out the services of another oncologist – one who took our concerns seriously.

Respect the time of your patients and their families

How many times were his doctors on time? Only once, during an illness that has spanned more than a year and scores of office visits.

Not once did a doctor or staff member call to say he or she was running late. And if I asked to use a phone while I waited so that I could do some of my own work, I was directed to the pay phone. Today, more physicians realize that their patients and their families have important lives, too. Their staffs call patients as soon as they know they are running late. And the most knowledgeable of them now equip their offices with phones for the convenience of their patients and their families.

Phone etiquette is important

When marketing and public relations consultants train physicians' office personnel in telephone etiquette, we usually concentrate on the staff. I now think this may be a mistake.

Although physicians' staffs were often rude on the phone, none were nearly as curt as the physicians themselves. Several doctors told us to feel free to call them or to have them paged at any time. The only problem with this arrangement was that when we did call them, they were usually busy and made it clear that our calls were an interruption. Remember, your patients' time is important, too. Don't make them feel by your tone of voice that they have inconvenienced you.

Set aside time during both the day and evening to return calls. Try not to make your patients feel like intruders. Brusqueness is never acceptable.

Don't be condescending

Condescension on the part of a doctor is not warranted. Treating patients badly could result over time in an empty waiting room.

Physicians today are just beginning to realize that it is the simple human skills that were not emphasized in medical school – especially communication – that can make or break a private practice.

My experiences tell me that many physicians are still behind the times when it comes to mastering these skills. They may be surviving, although in spite of how they act, not because of it. But in years to come, with their colleagues and competitors becoming more aware of marketing and public relations, physicians will have to become more adept in how they treat patients.

Julia E Schopick

"Take two aspirin and call me in the morning"

"Take two aspirin and call me in the morning." That standard piece of medical advice has worked so well that, abetted by television commercials showing people suffering horribly and seeking "adult-strength" preparations to bring "instant relief," the public collectively swallows hundreds of tons of acetylsalicylic acid (ASA) tablets to rid itself of assorted aches and pains and fevers.

This first of the so-called wonder drugs is easily available, cheap compared with other medications – and it works. But it's also an extremely potent substance.

Aspirin's heritage is simple enough: its principal element, salicylate, comes from the bark of the willow tree (salix), whose curative properties have been known for centuries; and ASA was first put together as a chemical compound in 1853. Scientists still are not quite sure exactly how the drug's analgesic action works. ASA's effectiveness in quickly bringing down high body temperatures is more clearly understood: it works on the central heat-regulating mechanism, and makes you sweat.

Because of its potency and complexity, ASA should be looked upon as something more than just a simple household remedy. It should be treated with respect, and used with discretion.

Quite apart from the fact that ASA is now the major cause of accidental poisoning in children, its side effects in people who take it knowingly – and even in quite small amounts – can be worse than the headache they set out to cure.

The main side effect is actually rather central – in the stomach. A couple of tablets of ASA have enough irritating acid to cause generally harmless gastric bleeding, but prolonged or repeated use may damage the stomach lining. People with ulcers should be extremely cautious about using the drug.

Some people, notably asthmatics, are particularly sensitive to ASA. It can cause dyspepsia, heartburn, skin eruptions, and a variety of other upsets, including "ringing in the ears." Fifty tablets – fewer in children – are enough to kill you if taken over a short period.

There are five main types of ASA: the straight, non-brand-name tablets; the sweetened, lower-dose children's version; the enteric-coated type released in the intestine and not in the stomach; the bubbling seltzer form which also contains antacids; and the combination tablet in which the ASA is mixed with codeine or other ingredients.

ASA gets into the bloodstream within 15 minutes, and half of it is excreted in the urine within less than 24 hours. As the advertisements say, it does indeed go to work quickly to relieve fever and pain. It is also effective in treating gout and rheumatoid arthritis. Contrary to popular opinion, it will not, however, cure your cold. But it will deaden some of the pain that accompanies it.

The shrill claims made by advertisers of the many competing forms of ASA preparation are enough to bring on a headache in themselves. Which to buy? Those that are "not recommended for children"? Those with seven grains instead of five? The ones that appear to transform, within seconds, the most hangdog expressions into surprised and delighted euphoria?

When properly used in appropriate dosages and for the proper indications, the least expensive, plain ASA will provide just as much relief, just as fast, for just as long a time, and with just the same side effects as the most expensive combination.

Other ASA watchers suggest that taking this stripped-down version of the drug with a little milk can help to alleviate stomach irritation.

ASA is a useful stand-by for relieving occasional minor problems. It's a marvellous drug, but it's often overused – and, occasionally, dangerous. Take two, certainly. But not too often. And if that headache persists, don't forget to call in the morning.

David Woods

Seven ways to build trust with your patients on their first visit

As a physician, you know that patient compliance is important to successful medical care. You hope your patients will follow your treatment plans, fill their prescriptions, and take their medication as directed. However, according to one US survey, physicians on average believe that as few as 62% of their patients are fully compliant. In surveys conducted elsewhere, this percentage has been as low as 46%. Patient compliance starts not in the exam room, but in the very first contact a new patient has with your office. How this first interaction develops is very often key to how much your patients will benefit from your treatment plans, so it is in your and your patients' best interests not to underestimate the important role your staff can play in developing compliance.

Many medical office staff say they no longer have the time to spend with patients that they used to enjoy. Cutbacks, reduced hours, and a more demanding patient base have all but eliminated the important "getting to know you" time that is so necessary to running a successful practice. To enhance the benefits of every patient visit, especially new-patient visits, nothing can be left to chance. The first meeting needs to be planned carefully by physicians and their staff.

1   *Scheduling*. New patients should, if possible, be scheduled for the least busy times of the day, and asked to come in ten minutes before their appointment time.
2   *Welcoming*. The patient should be greeted warmly by the receptionist or other specially designated staff people, who should tell the new patient their names and positions.
3   *Informing*. Once the introductions are over, the staff should then explain any procedures for this and future visits, such as providing a reason for the visit at the time of making the appointment, and the importance of bringing a health card or a list of medications. As often as possible, the staff should mention the doctor's name, such as: "Dr Morton needs to know the reason for your visit so we can book the right amount of time for your appointment," or "Dr Morton needs to know if you are taking any medication not prescribed by her, so whenever you come in, please bring a list of all medications you are taking."
4   *Collecting patient data*. New patients need to know from the very beginning that you and your staff respect the confidential nature of their relationship with you. Personal information should never be taken orally in a crowded reception room.
5   *Hosting the patient to the exam room*. Many doctors like to greet new patients in the reception area, but whether taking the patient to the exam room is done by staff or the doctor, this is an ideal time to solidify the relationship with the patient.

6   *Meeting the doctor.* Ideally, the first visit with the doctor will be more of an introductory meeting – the beginnings of establishing rapport – than treatment of an urgent medical problem, though in many cases, an urgent problem may be what has brought the patient there in the first place. If this is the case, the doctor should deal with the problem and ask the patient to book another appointment, when medical history and past treatments can be discussed in more detail.

7   *Saying goodbye.* This step involves patients with both doctor and staff. The medical component of the visit is over, and the patients are on the way out. You want them to leave feeling good about your practice, and to feel confident that they have found a physician who not only provides excellent medical care, but also runs an efficient office. Walking them out while saying goodbye provides a few moments to thank them, using their names, for choosing you as their doctor.

David Woods

Watch your language

Medicine and the English language

Language is a vital part of the therapeutic process. Yet aside from the often impenetrable prose of the social scientists, and the impeded monosyllables of the captive dental patient, medicine is perhaps the leading perpetrator of what Edwin Newman, author of *Strictly Speaking and A Civil Tongue*, jokingly calls "language viability destruction-generating capacity."

Obscurity, obliqueness, and jargon have for centuries hindered the therapeutic process: medical communication all too often confuses rather than enlightens. Maybe this is because medicine – although obviously becoming rapidly less so – is still an inexact science, its vagueness often reflected in its language.

A cartoon showing a patient strapped to a bed, hooked up to all manner of machinery and surrounded by a crowd of medical technologists, one of whom is saying: "We'd like to explain it to you in laymen's language, but we don't know any laymen's language," illustrates the point.

Doctors have long hidden behind jargon. The medieval physician Arnold of Villanova suggested that his 13th-century colleagues mask scientific ignorance with gobbledygook. When stuck for an answer, he advised, physicians should say that the patient has an obstruction of the liver, "and particularly use the word obstruction," he said, "because patients do not know what it means."

Physician/novelist Michael Crichton calls this, not quite wisely, obligatory obfuscation. In an article in the *New England Journal of Medicine*, he noted that among doctors this cannot be due to defensiveness because "while articles in medical journals may often be stuffy, stodgy, weak and equivocal, dense, impenetrable, and forbidding, physician-authors who are criticized in the letters columns of those same journals invariably respond in strong, brisk, and often stinging sarcastic prose."

Revealing that he is not immune to jargon himself, Crichton concluded that "medical obscurity may now serve an intragroup recognition function, rather like a secret fraternal handshake." This, he says, leads to those outside the charmed group having a low opinion of doctors.

Is there any cure for the chronic case of jargon that many physicians suffer from? Well, to start with, a more liberal education might help, if not exactly more Gray's *Elegy* than *Gray's Anatomy* then at least some literature and communications woven into the medical school curriculum.

Second, refusal by patients to be fobbed off with language they don't understand – just because they might be afraid of looking foolish.

Third, doctors might profitably mix with people other than doctors. Their social lives do tend to be confined to other medical folk – so the jargon becomes contagious.

In some instances when physicians had temporarily abandoned the scalpel for the pen they actually made the latter instrument seem more lethal. Among some of the horrors unearthed by one medical journal editor: "performing a postmortem on a dead person"; "in solo practice on my own"; "prostatectomy on a male"; and "per diem a day."

The English language is rich in eponym, something the dictionary defines as "a person, real or imaginary, from whom a tribe, place, institution, etc., takes, or is supposed to take, its name . . ." In the language of therapeutics eponyms abound. There's Braille, Bunsen, Mesmerize – and hundreds of diseases, tests, and syndromes named for their discoverers. Under the As alone there's Abrami's disease, Addison's, Albarran's, Alzheimer's, Albert's, Albright's, and half a dozen others.

For those no longer in need of medicine, we have Derrick (after a 17th-century hangman), and guillotine from Dr Guillotin – a humanitarian French physician who arguably alleviated more suffering than many of his professional colleagues before or since.

The language of medicine and therapeutics has also seeped into everyday speech. Hectic, chronic, and allergic are now no longer necessarily associated with medical matters – as in "he's allergic to work." And psychiatry has given us ambivalent, complex, inhibition, introvert, extrovert, masochistic, moron, phobia, and trauma.

Those who call for an end to jargon and obscurity can sometimes be guilty of both. The *New Yorker* once gleefully reported a newspaper paragraph that read: "Not being convinced, however, that theoretical lucidity is necessarily enhanced by terminological ponderosity, we shall avoid as much as possible the use of the sort of jargon for which both sociologists and phenomenologists have acquired dubious notoriety." The *New Yorker*'s question, quite rightly, was "When do you start?"

Practically everywhere, the language is in a mess. Police departments talk about "carrying out crime and punishment"; there are "fatal slayings" and "self-inflicted suicides"; there is "precipitation," never rain or snow. There is the persistently wrong use of "hopefully"; there's the non-existent "prestigious"; there's "between you and I." Viable, thereby, uptight, utilize, and "into" – as "I'm into better English" – have indeed been slain to death fatally, and should be allowed to rest.

As should the cliché, the packaged platitude in which so much communication appears these days. Is it too much to hope that something or somebody was last *and* least; that we could separate part from parcel, find people with no method in their madness, and who lack either rhyme or reason – but not both; and leave at least one stone unturned – and most commonplaces, banalities, and truisms overturned in favor of something more original.

James Thurber has said we "have become satisfied with gangrenous repetitions of threadbarisms . . . and the onset of utter meaninglessness is imminent." Medical science has done much for humanity, Thurber believed, but not in the area of verbal communication. He urged a prefectomy – cutting off the semi from semiprivate; the sub from subclinical, for a start. After all, said he, there must be a better way than "semiprivate" to describe a hospital room in which there are two or more beds.

Perhaps that humorist's solution to all this is the best one yet. Go and see what is called a "psychosemanticist" to straighten out any linguistic ailments you might suffer from.

But in the absence of such a desirable specialist, what can be done about language in therapeutics; about jargon, clichés, and inflated prose? About pomposity and obscurity?

The medical profession has, after all, produced a Somerset Maugham, a Conan Doyle, a Chekhov, and an Oliver Goldsmith, a Peter Roget and an AJ Cronin. What a stunning contribution by physicians to language and literature.

Unfortunately, there's a widespread feeling that to communicate well you must pad or disguise: weather forecasters are never content with showers, they must always say "shower activity"; "labour force participation" has replaced "work," and filing clerks have become "information retrieval operatives."

In the interests of fuller communication among different sciences, simplicity is vital. For example, "chlorophyll makes food by photosynthesis" isn't bad; but "green leaves build up food with the help of light" is even better. Sir Arthur Quiller-Couch, in his book *On The Art of Writing*, devoted a chapter to verbiage. He took the sentence, "In the case of John Jenkins, deceased, the coffin provided was of the usual character," and pulled it apart. It is superfluous to say that Jenkins is deceased; the fact that he needs a coffin is evidence enough. "In the case of" is also superfluous, for Jenkins did not have a case; he had, and needed, only a coffin. That coffin was not "of the usual character" since coffins have no character. The amended sentence read: "John Jenkins was provided with the usual coffin." One could have gone further and buried, along with Jenkins, the passive voice, but you get the point.

And language is – or should be – fun; not something to be swallowed like castor oil. Maybe that's what's wrong with the way it's taught in high schools – it's too threatening. And we can all of us respond critically to the abuse of language. We can, and should, draw attention to sloppy journalism; return incomprehensible memos; question garbled or conflicting advice; and hoot when people say renumeration.

One definition of news – an account of the differences between the world yesterday and the world today – might also apply to medicine where, figuratively at least, the differences between yesterday and today are enormous. Getting that information across is therefore important. And yet there seems to be a lack of agreement about how best to do it.

Why are physicians so modest about committing their knowledge to paper, and submitting it to the medical journals? Perhaps it's a linguistic diffidence that applies to most scientists. They're scared of appearing pushy and self-promoting.

Yet medical editors are delighted to receive a reasonably sound manuscript. They are not looking for works of literary genius. As medicine becomes increasingly complex, and medical knowledge and techniques expand at a frightening pace, it becomes ever more vital that doctors share their knowledge and experience with their colleagues. "What I've Learned" or "How I Do It" are much too important to be kept to yourself. Medical journal editors are interested in the practical, helpful presentation of down-to-earth medical information to busy people. As a putative author, you shouldn't feel that in order to appear learned you must write "This author is of the opinion that" when you simply mean "I think." And nobody will be particularly impressed if you write "At this time" when you mean "Now." So keep it simple. Be kind to the readers. And don't try to pull the wool over their eyes: if you say "It has long been known that . . ." the skeptic may feel that what you really mean is that you haven't bothered to look up the original reference but . . .

Similarly, a statement that something "is of wide-ranging theoretical and practical importance" may simply be taken to mean that you, the author, find it interesting. Another pitfall: "it is widely believed that . . ." cries out for credible reference. And if none is forthcoming, the reader may have the notion that Dr Jones down the corridor happens to share your point of view.

Robert Frost was right when he said that half the world is composed of people who have something to say and can't, and the other half of people who have nothing to say and keep on saying it. But then, another Robert – Benchley – thought the world was also divided into two groups: those who divide the world into two groups, and those who don't.

In any event, in the world today English is spoken by over 400 million people – more than speak any other of the world's 3000 or so languages except Mandarin Chinese. Certainly in therapeutics, as everywhere else, we can no longer afford obscurity, blandness, vagueness, and jargon.

Language is vital to the entire therapeutic process; but therapy seems to be increasingly necessary for our language.

David Woods

The printed word: encouraging a more coherent view of the world

"It is astonishing," wrote Sir William Osler, "with how little reading a doctor may practice medicine, but it is not astonishing how badly he may do it."

Since Osler's time the status and even the future of print have been threatened by radio, television, and audio and video cassettes, yet the printed word has endured and even prospered.

Neil Postman, professor of communication arts and sciences at New York University, stated in his book *Amusing Ourselves to Death: public discourse in the age of show business* that television will overwhelm words with pictures. Postman expresses a distinct preference for print, pointing out that the process of reading encourages rationality. He says that a printed page containing a narrative or argument that unfolds line by line encourages a more coherent view of the world than does a slambang broadcast of quickly changing, high-impact images.

Perhaps of more interest to physicians – members of a profession accustomed to doing rather than to being done to – is Postman's notion that reading is active, requiring the discipline of bodily stillness and mental attention, whereas watching television is essentially passive. Even if television were to vanish, the people of today who read almost nothing would still read almost nothing or would read the sort of printed matter that would cause Johannes Gutenberg to regret his invention of movable type. Even one of the most successful US medical publications, *Medical Economics*, is alleged to read consistently at the level of grades eight to ten. As Doug Mueller, president of the Gunner-Mueller Clear Writing Institute, puts it: "The successful business magazines realize that even educated professional people prefer to get information without straining."

But if it is true that education has produced a vast population able to read but unable to distinguish what is worth reading, it may well be that straining, in a different sense of the word, is exactly what is needed: one needs to sift what's worthy of reading from what isn't.

David Woods

Writing and speaking painlessly

George Orwell, whose style was plain and spare, observed that any rules for clear expression – even the ones that he suggested in his famous essay *Politics and the English Language* – should be broken if they force one to say anything barbarous. Thus, when flight attendants urge their passengers to observe the No Smoking sign or, worse still, to adhere to it, it sinks in that imprecise language occurs when people don't think first about exactly what it is they want to say.

What often lies between what people want to say or write, and what they actually do say or write, is an inadequate grasp of language. This grasp can be tightened by reading great writing, the choice of which is obviously a very subjective one, but Graham Greene, Somerset Maugham, and, of course, Orwell will do nicely if one's purpose is to learn and adopt clarity and simplicity.

In his book *How to Speak, How to Listen*, Mortimer Adler offers some tips on topics to be avoided in conversation, and which, if adopted universally, would enhance the social lives of millions. They are: one's state of health or recent surgical operation; one's babies and their cute little tricks; one's children and their brilliant accomplishments; and one's domestic pet, unless it happens to be an elephant, an alligator, or a boa constrictor.

Adler names three factors in persuasive speaking: ethos, pathos, and logos. Ethos consists in establishing the speaker's credibility and credentials; pathos consists in arousing the passions of the listeners and getting their emotions running in the direction of the action to be taken; and logos is the marshaling of reasoning.

Americans' number one fear is public speaking and, quite apart from potential hazards to an audience, the protagonist suffers in varying degrees from palpitations, dry mouth, wobbly knees, shaking hands, sweaty brow, and Niagaran armpits. Psychologically, the fear is of "drying up," and above all of looking foolish before one's fellow human beings. A group of researchers, in an experiment reported in the *Lancet*, hitched up electrocardiogram (ECG) monitors to 30 people speaking in front of audiences and recorded heart rates of up to 180 beats per minute. The researchers, who were perhaps relieved to present their findings in print rather than in person, noted that the intensity and nature of the individual speaker's reactions depend upon his personality, experience and health, the subject of the talk – and the audience.

The *Lancet* article showed the ECG reading for an "experienced and confident" speaker, a 27-year-old doctor addressing a medical meeting. At 5:23 p.m. his heart rate was 85; at 5:28 he began his speech and the rate shot up to 165; at 5:45 it was slower but still clipping along at 125. When he ended the talk at 5:55 his heart rate was back to 90, but it bounced back up to 110 at 6:00 when he was asked an "awkward question." The *Lancet* didn't say what that question was, but one hopes that after 32 minutes of stifled curiosity it might have been something like, "What are you doing with all those wires sticking out of your chest?"

The late Dr Ralph Smedley, founder of Toastmasters' International, urged prospective speakers to remember that their audience is just a group of individuals: "An audience of a hundred people is made up of individuals, any one of whom you can talk with individually. Talk to the group as one person." One of Smedley's successors, Maurice Forley, in his book *Public Speaking Without Pain*, reminds public speakers that they have, after all, been invited to speak and, if they know their material, know themselves, and know the audience, there is a reasonable chance that all will go well.

Those clear-eyed, firm-handshaking folk who run the Dale Carnegie courses earn their living by making those unaccustomed to public speaking less so. They contend that the fear of public speaking often starts in school, where red-faced kids are stood up in front of giggling, taunting classmates and towering, disapproving teachers to present an oral report. They believe that since nobody can escape having butterflies in the stomach, the best they can hope to do is to get them to fly in formation. The Carnegie technique is to convene a group of adults, each of whom is required to stand up and speak extemporaneously on a subject with which he is familiar. Mortimer Adler's advice to speakers is to use detailed notes rather than a complete text. Not everyone would agree. William F Buckley, Jr, one of North America's most accomplished orators and debaters, says in his book *Overdrive*: "My own feeling is that a proper speech should be polished, and to which end I tend to write mine out." Winston Churchill apparently had the best of both worlds – writing his speeches out completely, but telling them with all kinds of hesitancy and repetitions built in.

The successful writer tells people what they know already but haven't been able (or haven't dared) to put into words, and leaves it at that.

Orwell's *Politics and the English Language* is among the most widely cited of all 20th-century essays on the language, its central point being that sloppy language makes for sloppy thinking. In that essay, Orwell wrote that the battle against bad English is not frivolous and is not the exclusive concern of professional writers. He refers to the mixture of vagueness and sheer incompetence that is the most marked characteristic of modern English prose – which he says consists less and less of words chosen for the sake of their meaning, and more and more of phrases tacked together like the sections of a prefabricated henhouse. He warns against worn-out metaphors like having no axe to grind or having grist to the mill; he of course mentions mixed metaphors, giving as an example "the Fascist octopus has sung its swan song"; he urges avoiding the passive voice and such noun constructions as "by examination" instead of the gerund "by examining." Parenthetically, *Webster's Dictionary* uses as an example of the gerund: "Writing is easy." The example may be correct; the contention decidedly is not. And anyway, Orwell calls for eliminating phrases such as "having regard to" and "in view of," and for avoiding such foreign phrases as "status quo," unless there's absolutely no English equivalent.

Above all, Orwell calls for sincerity, simplicity, and concreteness. The great enemy of clear language, he says, is insincerity. He suggests that political language consists largely of euphemism, question begging, and cloudiness. For example: "Defenceless villages are bombarded from the air, the inhabitants driven out into the countryside, the cattle machine-gunned, the huts set on fire with incendiary bullets – this is called pacification."

Orwell gives in the essay a wonderful example of the decay of the language. He starts by quoting a well-known verse from Ecclesiastes: "I returned and saw under the sun, that the race is not to the swift, nor the battle to the strong, neither yet bread to the wise, nor yet riches to men of understanding, nor yet favour to men of skill; but time and chance happeneth to them all." He translates this into modern English as follows: "Objective consideration of contemporary phenomena compels the conclusion that success or failure in competitive activities exhibits no tendency to be commensurate with innate capacity, but that a considerable element of the unpredictable must invariably be taken into account."

David Woods

Who's for Tennyson?
The case for language and
literature in medical school

In his impious 1911 glossary *The Devil's Dictionary*, Ambrose Bierce defined a physician as "one upon whom we set our hopes when ill and our dogs when well."

But in today's medicine, our hopes are more likely to rest with an array of sophisticated technologies and gadgetry, rather than with a human being. Dr Jerry Vannatta, former dean of the University of Oklahoma College of Medicine, says: "This technology has become a religion within the medical community. It is easy to lose sight of the fact that still, in the 21st century . . . 80 to 85 percent of the diagnosis is in the patient's story."

Yet many physicians today lack either the skill, the time, or the inclination to listen to that story – a talent that used to be called bedside manner. This is a shame because of the four elements in communication – speaking, reading, writing, and listening – listening is learned first, is used most through life, and is taught least through all the years of schooling. Yet deficiencies in listening and the ensuing failures of communication are a major source of wasted time, ineffective operation, miscarried plans, and frustrated decisions. In medicine, they can also be a source of error and litigation.

But according to the *New York Times*, "It is this lost art of listening to the patient that has been the inspiration behind a burgeoning movement in medical schools throughout the country: Narrative Medicine." This is part of a growing trend toward exposing medical students to the humanities.

Narrative Medicine's founder, Dr Rita Charon, teaches such a course at Columbia University's medical school. In the 19th century, she says, doctors carefully and humbly visited with patients and listened to them, and not just with a stethoscope.

Parenthetically, the inventor of that instrument, RT Laennec, required *his* medical students to take exhaustive notes after seeing a patient. Dr Charon believes that medicine has been struggling to come close to the patient ever since that time. "Medicine," she says, "is beholden to the singular experience of individual patients; we've always known this. But it's been eclipsed by a heady optimism that because we understand organ systems and molecular biology we understand the patient."

"If you listen to patients' lament," she says, "it's not that 'my doctor can't open my stent'; it's that 'my doctor doesn't listen to me'." Not that Dr Charon has much time for bland exhortations to create a more caring and empathic medical profession. "What's needed," she says, "is the prescription; the How."

And that's what Narrative Medicine is about: reading, writing, perceiving – paying attention. Since 1982, Dr Charon's students have been analyzing in literary terms that which they hear and read. It has to do with eliciting nuance and subtlety.

She emphasizes that this is no soft option course. Not only are Columbia medical students required to take graduate-level humanities courses, the material itself is presented in a highly rigorous and disciplined manner. Says Dr Charon, who is an internal medicine physician who also has a doctorate in English: "When I teach Henry James here, I do so as I would in the English Department."

Dr Charon's group also produces a semi-annual journal, *Literature and Medicine*, which is published by Johns Hopkins University Press; and Oxford University Press will publish her book *Narrative Medicine: honoring the source of illness*. To further its objectives, Columbia's course features a writer-in-residence – currently Susan Sontag, author of *Illness As Metaphor*.

Another well-known exponent of communication skills for medical students was the late Norman Cousins. Cousins, who wrote *Anatomy of an Illness*, the story of his diagnosis and treatment for ankylosing spondylitis, was an eminent journalist who went on to teach medical students at UCLA. In an interview with him some years ago (*see* pp. 43–7), he told me that he'd developed a survey of 500 patients. One of the questions was: "If you've ever changed doctors – why?" "That really got the attention of the students," he recalled.

Cousins went on to say that "What is required [of a doctor] is the deepest possible understanding of what the patient is talking about. Respect for the patient." His survey yielded such responses as "He was a very competent physician but he really didn't know what my problem was" or "I admired him as a doctor but I had no confidence in him as a human being." Cousins' conclusion was that it is the *style* of the physician, not the competence of the physician, that is the yardstick people use for keeping or changing their doctors.

Cousins further believed that "medicine begins with science but treatment of human beings involves artistry. Physicians need to marry art to science." Moreover – shades of Narrative Medicine – Cousins told me that "novelists portray the physician not just as a prescriber of medicaments but as a symbol of all that is transferable from one human being to another."

All of this is not simply to create a new layer of kinder, gentler doctors – or to graft some Gray's *Elegy* onto *Gray's Anatomy*. It's to rediscover a fundamental part of the diagnostic and therapeutic process, one that will make the patient's medical encounter more productive and less frightening. "Doctorspeak" too often means jargon that's incomprehensible to patients, who may not be at their receptive or emotional best. And the impersonal "put the emphysema in the other ward and bring the prostate biopsy in here" doesn't help. Nor does the absolving "We" – also favored by royalty and editorial writers – as in "How are we, today?" or "We see a lot of that."

Novelist and psychologist Liam Hudson in *The State of the Language* says there is a "crisis of intelligibility" among scientists, and notes that the truth can best be grasped by prose that is itself vigorous, disciplined, and plain. Noting that scientists are barely able to utter a sentence that does not include the key words *situation*, *interaction*, and *role*, Hudson says that by contrast the business of writing a novel or a poem is one of highly-wrought discipline. "What lies between scientists and their subject matter," he says, "is an inadequate grasp of the English language. Their grasp can be tightened by reading, interpreting – and understanding – the great writers."

Tennyson, anyone?

David Woods

Splitting atoms and infinitives

Physicians, more than any other professionals except perhaps lawyers, live by the word, yet their lengthy education contains little or no specific instruction in the design and management of language.

This is a pity, because scientists are among the few who have anything brand new to tell us. But, too often, they refrain from doing so because they don't know *how* to tell us. Is this because the scientist is a perfectionist, and therefore loath to become involved in the uncertainties, nuances, and lack of formula in language? Is the person who split the atom afraid to tell us in case, in so doing, he splits an infinitive?

Quite possibly you may feel that what you're doing isn't earth shattering enough to justify its publication; that medical practice is pretty dull and routine. You may even think that only heart transplants, breakthroughs, miraculous cures, and oracular pronouncements merit publication. Or, more possibly, you still believe that the only real research is done by groups of white-coated technicians working behind closed doors.

And yet, to a greater or lesser degree, all physicians are researchers; how often do you, for instance, tell a fellow physician of some new or interesting discovery you have made? The problem lies in persuading doctors to capture the content of corridor consultations, and commit it to writing for the benefit of a wider audience.

Doctors who have something to say should share their knowledge and experience with their colleagues; indeed, they have an obligation to do so. Never mind the grammar: logic and content are what matter most in getting your facts across. The cardinal sin in medical writing is not grammatical error, but obscurity.

Physicians, whether they've spent 40 years in practice or have just completed their first 24 hours, have experiences to report. Yet, oddly enough, the "publish or perish" epidemic that swept over a whole generation of researchers and academics seemed to leave doctors largely unaffected.

The reason for this is not altogether clear, but it may have to do with what one teacher calls the need to develop a "conceit" among physicians; a realization that what they have to say is worth listening to. And so it is.

Perhaps physicians who want to share valuable knowledge or experience are inclined to procrastinate: to persuade themselves that they don't really have the time, to worry about the possibility of their manuscripts being rejected, or to rely on the old "I know it but I don't know how to write it" excuse.

A curious attitude characterizes physicians' approach to writing. This is perhaps typified by the doctor who, on being introduced to an author, said: "When I retire, I too intend to write books." The author replied: "Tremendous; when I retire, I'm going to become a neurosurgeon."

Writing does indeed take time and effort, but what you have to say probably can't be put off until you have limitless leisure time to write it down. Nor, given that you really have something to say, does it have to be brilliantly written. Medical editors become almost human when they receive unsolicited scientific manuscripts whose content is worthwhile.

So long as submitted material has facts, logic, and form, most editors are quite happy to overlook its literary shortcomings. Indeed, there is something of a challenge in turning a stodgy treatise into readable form.

If you have something worthwhile to tell other doctors, make the time to put it in writing. Don't worry too much about how it's written – that's what editors are for. They'll do any surgery that may be necessary on your dangling participles.

David Woods

Making sure your language doesn't mystify patients

Common words are learned faster and remembered longer. Thus, word frequency is a good estimate of word difficulty: common (easy) words show up more frequently in written materials; uncommon (hard) words show up less frequently. The *Word Frequency Guide* (Brewster, NY: Touchstone Applied Science Associates) identifies some common (easy) and uncommon (hard) words in three report cards:

Frequency per million words

10 000	a, and, for, in, of, on, that, the, too
3000	about, if, from, not, people, their, will
1000	also, been, its, important, make, than, those, use
300	among, example, information, keep, members, public
100	available, current, differences, particular, report, results, services
30	appropriate, approximately, extremely, factors, indicates
10	access, assurance, barriers, comparisons, graph, meaningful, survey
3	assessing, inappropriate, options, specialty, statistical, utilization
< 1	accredited, affiliated, carefulness, color-coded, demographic, ensuring, inconvenience, provider, respondents

Patients may be able to read the words in report cards – they just don't know what they mean. "Utilization" shows up three times in every million words; "use" shows up 1000 times in every million words; "approximately," 30 times per million words, but "about," 3000 times per million words. Your ability to communicate with your patients has much more effect than the statistics in a report card. Make sure that your patients are not mystified by your words.

Mark Hochhauser

Reforming the language of healthcare

The word "patient" means suffering or enduring without complaint. Until recently, it has been an apt name for the person who comes to you for treatment.

But that's changing. As Regina Herzlinger puts it in *Market-Driven Health Care*, we are entering a healthcare age in which hour-long waits, fragmented care, red tape, and inconvenient locations will give way to customer-focused, convenient, courteous, informative, and easy-to-use products and services. "Well-informed, mastery-seeking [patients]," she says, "are no longer going to put you or anybody else up on a pedestal. Make them your partner, not your enemy, in the healthcare process."

Perhaps these partners, accustomed to being wooed and cosseted in all the other transactions they make, are becoming impatient – a case, if ever there was one, for replacing the word "patient." In *The Devil's Dictionary*, Ambrose Bierce defines patience as "a minor form of despair, masquerading as a virtue."

Yet a study of 308 outpatients at one Australian hospital concluded that four out of five respondents preferred the term "patient" to "client" or "customer." A letter writer in the *British Medical Journal* suggested that in this egalitarian age both doctors and patients be referred to as "actors;" another writer, tongue firmly in cheek, proposed that in this litigation-happy era we might simply change titles from "doctor" and "patient" to "defendant" and "plaintiff." Still others have called for "user," but this has negative – not to mention narcotic – overtones.

"Patron" has a nice ring to it. Physicians and patrons. And while we're in the business of reforming the language of medicine, let's dispense with that dreadful word "provider," which makes doctors sound like merchants. And now that we've got rid of "patient," isn't it time to abandon "waiting room" in favor of "reception area"?

David Woods

Euphemism in medicine: calling a spade a horticultural implement

A school board wanted to ban Shakespeare's *The Merchant of Venice* because it views the bard's depiction of Shylock, the Jewish moneylender, as antisemitic; the South African government banned Anna Sewell's children's classic *Black Beauty* because of its title; and the Inner London Education Authority ordered that Beatrix Potter's *Peter Rabbit* and *Benjamin Bunny* be removed from schools under its jurisdiction because the stories concern only "middle-class rabbits."

How happy Thomas Bowdler would be with all of this. After years spent in medicine, travel, and philanthropy, and some study of the education of children, Bowdler set out in 1818 to "purify" the works of Shakespeare, striking from them "those words and expressions ... which cannot with propriety be read aloud in a family." The word "bowdlerize" was first used in print in 1836 and became a term of abuse, although the process of expurgation that it represents is clearly still with us.

Physician–author Richard Asher believed that hedging, fudging, and euphemism are very much a part of medicine. Describing the modern hematologist, Asher referred to him as someone who "instead of describing in English what he can see, prefers to describe in Greek what he can't."

Asher went on to say that if physicians don't know something, they don't admit it; instead, they try to confuse their listeners by using what he called "medspeak." One such smokescreen, Asher said, involves the physician's abandoning plain English "in an attempt to appear learned, 'upbeat', or succinct and, in the process, to hide. In these circumstances, one's 'communication' consists of long words, jargon, abbreviation, and equivocation."

By definition, euphemism means substitution of a favorable for a more accurate but possibly offensive expression. Literally, it means fair of speech. Thus, there are no longer any old people, only "senior citizens"; the poor have become "the underprivileged"; drug addicts are "the chemically dependent"; and children of low intelligence are "exceptional students." And people do not die: they "pass away." When they do, they are ministered to not by an undertaker but by a "mortician"; their burial plot is merely a "place of rest," prepared not by a gravedigger but by an "interment engineer."

Euphemisms have been referred to as verbal placebos. Theodore M Bernstein says that "euphemisms are not fig leaves, intended to hide something; they are diaphanous veils, intended to soften grossness or starkness."

The danger in all this – in medicine and elsewhere – is that euphemism leads to obscurity and misunderstanding. Surely we and our language are mature enough nowadays to call a spade a spade, not a horticultural implement.

David Woods

Humor in medicine: the whimsy of Richard Gordon

Medicine has been described as one of the gloomy professions. Yet author Norman Cousins believes that humor is a marvellous antidote to what ails you, and author Richard Gordon (*Doctor in the House*, *Doctor at Sea*, *Doctor at Large*, etc.) has written dozens of books on humor in medicine.

Gordon began his writing career preparing obituary notices for the *British Medical Journal*, an activity that he describes as a superb training for a writer of fiction, although, in fact, his first book was a text on anesthetics and is still in print.

Although the "Doctor" books were hugely successful, and many of them were turned into movies in which such actors as Brigitte Bardot and the late Sir Kenneth More and Sir Dirk Bogarde performed, Gordon believes that critics – at least in his native England – tend to dismiss humorous literature. As an example, he cites one reviewer's comment on AA Milne: "He was a good writer if only a humorist."

Gordon thinks there are remnants of feudalism in British medicine today. A patient asking for a diagnosis is likely to be told "Don't worry. It has a long Latin name that you wouldn't understand." He says that he has an anxiety neurosis that worries him deeply, and, with a touch of black humor, he says that he would bring back the "Black Death" because that would be one way of solving the problem of overcrowding. Gordon is a self-confessed name-dropper who suffers from nominal aphasia. He is also a champion of the suburbs (he lives just outside of London) because, as he puts it, "You can live your own life there – the people are all so frightened of being thought suburban that no one talks to their neighbours." He peppers his speech with archaic Britishisms like "Jolly good!" and terms from cricket, a game he loves, like "sticky wicket."

On the alleged "downside" of scientific progress – Chernobyl, the space-shuttle disasters, acid rain, and so on – Gordon points out that the first steam locomotive ran over and killed a politician during its inaugural trip, which shows, in his view, that there can sometimes be benefits in disaster.

Noting that power is delightful and absolute power is absolutely delightful, Gordon says that if ever he attains it his first move will be to open the pubs all day. He enjoys a few pink gins every evening, a throwback to his days as a ship's doctor, which became the basis for the best-selling *Doctor at Sea*. It is perhaps fitting, although not at all funny, that this humorist suffers from one of the few diseases that evoke laughter, not pity – gout.

As for medicine being a gloomy profession, Gordon disagrees. He thinks it's a jolly profession. And he's certainly enjoyed great success in portraying it as such. Jolly good!

David Woods

Elevator etiquette: when is communication too effective?

Standing at the back of the hospital elevator, a hospital physician observed that on the second floor, two other physicians got on and began to discuss the patient they were seeing. Their discussion was so explicit that by the end of the ride, he notes, he could probably have taken care of that patient.

This experience will be familiar to many readers. Hospital employees treat elevators like just another place to get their work done. Physicians dictate patient notes, residents discuss intriguing cases, and nurses talk about hospital life without thinking about how this will affect other passengers.

Our eavesdropping doctor decided it was time to bring attention to this issue. He recruited a group of medical ethics students to eavesdrop on elevator conversations. He told them to dress in street clothes, so they would look like ordinary hospital visitors, and instructed them to write down any inappropriate comments made by hospital employees.

They not only heard breaches of patient confidentiality, but they also heard hospital employees talking about themselves in ways that raised questions about whether they could or wanted to provide quality care to their patients. A physician got on the elevator and complained to another that he was leaving his job as soon as possible so that he could go somewhere where he could make more money. Two administrators mentioned that the coroner had to be brought in on a case because the patient's death was the hospital's fault.

Many healthcare professionals do not do an effective job of communicating medical information to their patients. However, part of effective communication is knowing when and what not to communicate. The unedited comments overheard in these elevators are clearly an example of over-enthusiastic communication.

Almost every physician who has heard about this research says, "Oh, that's one of my pet peeves. Thanks for doing that study." It seems as if this is a sin that all are guilty of except ourselves.

Peter E Ubel MD

A conversation with Norman Cousins

In 1964, when he was 49, Norman Cousins, former editor of the respected American magazine *Saturday Review*, contracted ankylosing spondylitis; his physicians gave him one chance in 500 of recovering. In his book *Anatomy of an Illness* Cousins told how he surmounted these odds by using the unconventional combination of massive doses of vitamin C and even heftier amounts of positive thinking.

Working with his personal physician, Dr William Hitzig, Cousins set out to answer the question: is it possible that love, hope, faith, laughter, confidence, and the will to live have therapeutic value?

Cousins followed a systematic regime of *Candid Camera* classics, Marx Brothers movies, Elwyn Brook and Katharine White's *Subtreasury of American Humor*, and Max Eastman's *The Enjoyment of Laughter*. He made the "joyous discovery that ten minutes of genuine belly laughter had an anesthetic effect" and found that his astronomic erythrocyte sedimentation rate declined.

After an account of his illness was published in the *New England Journal of Medicine*, he received 3000 letters from physicians, most of them in support. Cousins was sufficiently encouraged to write a book. "One of the most striking features of these letters," he says, "is evidence of the new respect among doctors for the ideas of non-professionals." Cousins concludes that his own respect for the medical profession is undiminished.

Over his 40-year career Cousins carried out presidential missions abroad; acted as a personal emissary to Pope John XXIII in successfully negotiating the release of two cardinals from eastern European prisons; headed the project carrying out medical and surgical treatment for victims of the atomic bombing of Hiroshima; headed a similar program that provided medical care for victims of Nazi medical experimentation; organized a program that brought medicine and food to thousands of Biafran children; was one of the founders of public television in the United States; and headed the special task force that set up an environmental program in New York City.

After leaving the editorship of *Saturday Review*, he accepted an invitation to join the Faculty of Medicine at the University of California at Los Angeles, where he served as adjunct professor in the program of medicine, law, and human values. This interview was conducted by the then editor of the *CMAJ* and took place in Norman Cousins' office at UCLA.

You have called for an increasing infusion of the liberal arts into medical education. Yet the goal orientation of the people who are going to become physicians may be such that if the curriculum doesn't translate into something that will be asked of them in examinations or will be used in the very narrowest sense of traditional practice, it's difficult to weave into medical school. Courses in ethics and administration are examples. How can room be made for courses in language and communication?

When I came to UCLA I had very little success in talking to medical students. My physician colleagues have made me feel very much at home, but I did have a problem trying to get students' attention for these so-called soft subjects.

Because there was no pay off?

Yes, there was no way of quantifying it so how could they be sure they were going to get the right answer in examinations? And that's what counted. Also, I couldn't make the connection between what I was talking about and effective medical practice. So I decided that I would really have to go at them in terms of the bottom line. I developed a survey of 500 patients, being careful to make sure that these would be regarded as desirable patients by the doctors – people well educated, people of status in the communities, people whose recommendations would carry weight with other patients. A question I asked was: if you have ever changed doctors – why? That really got the attention of the medical students.

If physicians don't stroke and smooth patients, they are going to lose money?

If patients want to be stroked or smoothed they don't deserve to be treated. I mean that. What is required, however, is not stroking and smoothing but the deepest possible understanding of what the patient is talking about. Respect for the patient. Giving a patient some sense that the doctor knows what the patient is talking about. For instance, we received responses like: "He was a very competent physician but he really didn't know what my problem was." "I admired him as a doctor but I had no confidence in him as a human being." "He kept being interrupted by phone calls, would take these phone calls, or talk about things that had nothing to do with my case." So out of this awareness came the rather startling conclusion that it's the style of the physician, not the competence of the physician, that is the yardstick people use for keeping or changing their doctors.

What about the concept of unrealistic expectations?

Well, if I were a doctor with a big overhead and I had made up my mind about this particular patient and all the patient was doing was repeating, I'd get pretty damned impatient myself. But even allowing for that, I don't think nine minutes with the patient, especially in complex cases where the doctor has to make determinations and where technology can only carry him so far and where the cognitive function of the doctor is going to determine whether that diagnosis is correct, that that is enough time. Yet I know the doctor may say, well, with increases in rent, in salaries, in malpractice insurance premiums, "What do you want me to do, subsidize my patients? I can't afford to do that." But I think it's important for all of us to face up to the problem of communicating with patients.

Given your own experience with illness, what have you learned about the patient in the doctor–patient relationship?

The most striking thing I've observed is the tendency of patients with serious illness to go into a very severe and rapid intensification of their symptoms coincident with the diagnosis. I have met with some 262 cancer patients, most of whom will say that as soon as they left the doctor's office they discovered an acceleration of symptoms following the diagnosis.

In other words, when they hear they fear. Naming a disease exacerbates it?

Precisely. The moment a label is attached to their symptoms their bodies produce the kinds of effects that they had associated with that particular disease. The body follows the expectations. I'll give you an example. At a high school football game, four people reported ill at half-time. The examining physician ascertained that the only thing they had in common, other than that their symptoms were roughly identical – severe abdominal pains, dizziness, nausea – was that they had all consumed drinks from the same dispensing machine. An announcement was made telling people about the four and requesting that no one consume any soft drinks until the precise cause of the illness could be determined. The moment that announcement was made the stadium became a sea of retching and fainting people. Ambulances from five hospitals had to ply back and forth to pick up people with the same symptoms as those who had become ill. Hundreds of others went home to see their own doctors. When it was discovered that the drinks had nothing to do with the illness and that the four people had a purely coincidental experience, a further announcement was made at the stadium and in the hospitals. The people suddenly improved and their symptoms disappeared. Charcot's conversion hysteria. If people at a football game can become ill just because of suggestive sounds, patients who have the word "cancer" attached to their symptoms may find their life going that much faster down that road. It seems to me we use the term "iatrogenic" too restrictively to mean too much medication or the wrong medication, to apply to surgery when mistakes are made. But there is such a thing as iatrogenesis caused by poor communication.

Surely you would not suggest that the hysteria engendered at that football game would have a parallel with cancer?

Not the cause of cancer. But once the people knew, once they had a label to attach to their symptoms, and they had expectations of what cancer was, their bodies followed the expectations.

So how does communication influence the disease process?

Sounds can produce illness. Words, whether used in print or orally, can produce illness. During the Middle Ages thousands of people went dancing in the streets with the hysteria of St Vitus. But this dance and the illness were real. Hysteria, in whatever form, is illness, even though it may not be identifiable on a slide. Similarly, you had the disease tarantus in Italy, where many thousands of people were convinced they had been bitten by spiders and their symptoms were precisely as though they had been. The illness was real, though the spiders were not. People can become ill as a result of what they think and hear and see; and this would suggest that the physician's role in communicating with the patient is not merely important but central, basic, in treatment.

Would you then suggest that, while one might harness science to treat disease, the physician would be better off presenting a front of warmth and reassurance than one of definition and scientific terminology?

I'm not sure that there's a conflict between the physician as scientist and the physician as artist. I think that medicine begins with science but that treatment of human beings involves artistry. You apply science artistically. I think physicians need to marry art to science.

In fact, you've said in your books that the doctor is a powerful placebo.

I think that historically people have had to overcome dangerous treatment – bleeding, purging, and so on – but belief in the physician was the most powerful medication. As [Franz] Inglefinger [former editor of the New England Journal of Medicine] said: 85% of the illnesses from which people go to the doctors' offices are self-limiting and the doctor can help in that process. But some of them can become chronic if the communication suggests to the patient that this is not within easy reach. Panic is the great disease of our time. If doctors fail to liberate the patient from panic, they miss an important part of what the treatment has to be.

Yet the exigencies of medical practice are that an open-ended, overutilized, "free" healthcare system has created an assembly line for physicians, particularly family practitioners, many of whom would love to be able to take the patient by the hand – let's say the patient with anxiety – and counsel that patient. The practicality is that they prescribe tranquilizers instead. With increasingly sophisticated pharmacotherapy and technology, won't the very kind of time-consuming reassurance you advocate be militated against by the harsh reality of medical practice?

The evidence of that is in the 60 million prescriptions of tranquilizers in the United States each year. Connected with that, of course, is a question: if 85% of people who go to doctors' offices have no business being there, does this mean that 85% of them do not come away with prescriptions? Doctors have been educated by patients to provide prescriptions. If they don't, someone else will. It's too easy to give people tranquilizers. Of course, there are many cases where tranquilizers can make a profound difference in a person's life. But 60 million prescriptions?

Yet we live in a society in which we're used to pressing buttons and getting instant results. In disease, that creates an expectation that there's going to be an instant solution. People tend to say, "I've got something wrong with me, I want it fixed and I want it fixed now."

Yes, but it's not only a quick fix but an external fix. We think that with any illness the only way you can possibly get better is by reaching for something and pouring it into you. As medicine becomes increasingly specialized it becomes more and more externalized, and as it becomes more and more externalized the distance between patient and physician increases. Every time you go to a referral or to a diagnostic machine and then a referral beyond the diagnostic machine, you are increasing the distance between yourself and the doctor, who is such a powerful ingredient in helping set you right.

You said in *Anatomy of an Illness* that death is not the great tragedy, but depersonalization is.

I think that death is not the enemy but constant fear of dying is. I believe that people in North America have pushed it in the wrong direction by public health education. The effect of public health education in schools and on TV or radio programs, in the press and in advertising, is to make us rather panicky – very insecure about ourselves. It doesn't help to educate us about how human beings function. It doesn't give us confidence in ourselves. It doesn't enable us to make correlations between the pains we may have and the abuses to which we subject our body. It makes us into a nation of hypochondriacs and self-medicaters. On one hand you have "education" pushing people into insecurity and vulnerability, and then you have the advertising of quick nostrums – analgesics, sleeping pills, etc.

You have said that novelists portray the physician not just as a prescriber of medicaments but as a symbol of all that is transferable from one human to another, short of immortality. I assume you must favor the concept of the family physician who, ideally, treats the entire person in exactly the way you have been talking about. He knows you, your family, your history, your interests, your job, and all of those other things that influence one's well-being.

Yes – and who has enough background on you to recognize your panic as a principal factor, and who liberates you from it. He is able to say, "Joe, I want to tell you something. You've had a hard time at the office, you've had a hard time with the family, you haven't been able to sleep. As a result you might be overeating, or eating too rapidly. You're getting all these tensions in your life and your body is crying out in pain. I can give you some pills and quiet you down but I don't think you need them. You're intelligent enough to know the connection between what you're doing and what the effects are on your body. You've got to listen to what your body is trying to tell you, and I'm always here. If I'm wrong, you're going to let me know about this. But in the meantime just have confidence in yourself – you're alright, you're not diseased, you don't have cancer, you don't have heart disease."

Your own physician, Dr William Hitzig, to whom you dedicated your book *Human Options*, was very supportive of the approach you took to your own disease.

I have had very good luck with all my physicians. But I think it is very difficult to practice good medicine nowadays for the reasons I mentioned.

Does the public tend to glorify physicians, and to expect too much from them?

I think that the healing power of the physician comes as much from the belief in his curative powers as from all the medicines and facilities at his command.

You say the liberal arts have been downplayed in medical education and that medical students' scholastic energies tend to be focused in studies that deal with quantifiable matters. How do you achieve that broadening if you're going to train a professional who can deal with human beings from all walks of life?

I think that in the last few years we have seen a closer connection between the physician and society, certainly with respect to the total health of the society. I have been especially impressed with the development of organizations such as the Physicians for Social Responsibility. Here you have people in medicine who understand deeply that if you are concerned about the health of individuals you have to be concerned about those things that affect health in the large.

David Woods

The future of medical publishing

The following is the text of a speech given to the students and faculty at the University of the Sciences in Philadelphia in May 2004.

Commenting on the future of anything is a mixed blessing. On the one hand, for an editorialist it offers an irresistible combination of temptation and opportunity; on the other hand, one is mindful of the many who have upended themselves memorably on the banana peel of prediction.

For instance, in 1800, Thomas Malthus, a practitioner of what later became known as "the dismal science" of economics, famously foretold of a world population imminently to be extinguished by its inability to feed itself. Today, a senior fellow of the Hoover Institute claims that "the entire population of the world could be housed in the state of Texas, in single-story houses – four people to a house – and with a typical yard around each home."

This assumes, of course, that you could persuade them all to move to Texas.

In 1943, Thomas Watson, then-chairman of IBM, stated confidently that there was a world market for about five computers. And CP Scott, crusty editor of the (then *Manchester*) *Guardian* is said to have snorted: "Television? The word's half Greek and half Latin: no good can possibly come of it." No wonder Yogi Berra vowed that he would predict anything except the future.

What I'd like to try to do here is to offer some brief background and statistics, discuss the impact of managed care and electronic publishing, comment on international opportunities, trace some trends – and say why I believe that in this information age, an age of concurrently dwindling attention spans, there will always be a role in medical publishing for savvy and linguistically rigorous writers, editors and publishers.

Since Thomas Wakley published the first issue of the *Lancet* in 1823 – as he put it "to put an end to mystery and concealment" in the world of medicine – the sum total of medical knowledge has increased explosively (today there are some 25 000 biomedical journals) and the speed at which communication is achieved has been even more dramatic. In Wakley's time, the speed of communication was no faster than a human or a horse could carry it. Today's communication is about two-thirds of a billion miles per hour. The good news is that that's as fast as it *can* go. Unless, of course, Einstein was wrong.

The bad news is that costs have no such limitations. While Wakley's *Lancet* sold for sixpence, average annual subscription prices for medical periodicals surged from $51 in 1977 to a whopping average four-digit price in many instances today. No wonder Cornell University recently decided to review and severely prune the $1.7 million a year it was paying mega-medical publisher Elsevier for some 930 science journals.

In his book *The Inarticulate Society*, Tom Shachtman says that Americans today watch 1500 hours of television a year, which means about 50 days a year; or, if we extrapolate a bit, roughly nine years by the time they reach 65 if they haven't expired earlier from boredom. By contrast, they spend a combined total of only 290 hours reading newspapers and magazines. Part of this decline in literacy, says Shachtman, is the chasm between the literate-based and oral languages. He refers to a computerized scale of comprehension skill in which a "level of difficulty" of an article in a scientific journal, *Nature*, rates 58.6 units, compared with a sample of *Time* magazine at 6.8 and of *The National Enquirer* at *minus* 10.3. He then goes on to note that "knowledge derived from [print] tends to remain more detailed, to stay with us longer, and to be more broadly based than what we receive from television." Perhaps that's why the three principal medical television companies have ceased to exist in the past couple of years.

Neil Postman, professor of communications at New York University, points out that the process of reading encourages rationality. Postman – surely a felicitous eponym for the bearer of such an epistle – says that a printed page containing a narrative or argument that unfolds line by line encourages a more coherent view of the world than does a slambang broadcast of quickly changing, high-impact images.

Speaking of slambang images, you may have noticed that I have no PowerPoint. And it's not by any means because I believe that PowerPoint corrupts. Rather it's because I think that the modern Lancet is at least partly right – and not merely demonstrating some kind of journalistic arteriosclerosis – when in a recent issue it published an article titled "PowerPoint: Shot with its own bullets." That article invited readers to "Imagine a world with almost no pronouns or punctuation. A world where any complex thought has to be broken into seven-word chunks, with colorful blobs between them" . . . and where it's hard to accommodate full English sentences, so that meaning may be obscured.

In any event, there's a wonderful invention known as the Box Of Organized Knowledge. It has no electrical circuits or wires or mechanical parts, can be used anywhere, and consists of a number of sheets of paper bound together. The symbols on each sheet are absorbed optically and registered on the brain. This phenomenon is known by its acronym BOOK.

The *Economist*, in a special report on the future of medicine, noted that doctors are finding it hard to absorb ever more information, and that American doctors typically spend no more than three hours a week educating themselves. And for most of them, the report says, applying the knowledge gained from reading journals has become as much an art as a science. The information can often be conflicting and few doctors have any idea how to resolve such conflicts. Not that this is a new phenomenon. More than a century ago Sir William Osler noted: "It is astonishing with how little reading a doctor may practice medicine, but it is not astonishing how badly he may do it."

Although the term "information explosion" has already been relegated to the ranks of cliché, the issue it describes is still very much with us. According to Veronis, Suhler and Associates, a New York company that analyzes business trends in the communications industry, health science and business are still the two fastest growing subsets of the multibillion dollar US professional publishing and information sectors. The company noted the following trends:

- Mergers and acquisitions in the medical publishing industry will continue.
- Access to information will be a continuum – 24 hours a day, seven days a week.
- Constant updating of information will be vital.
- A move towards just-in-time publishing, and customized product packaging – even in print – will accelerate.
- Products on shelves will be marginalized as healthcare professionals increasingly seek information online.
- Medical journals rely heavily on libraries, associations, individual practitioners – and pharmaceutical advertising. Spending in this category is $628 million, but will decelerate as publishers adopt online content, a move driven by increasing demand for solutions-oriented publishing.
- VS forecasts that total spending on *all forms* of healthcare media will rise at an annual rate of 7%, hitting $4.8 billion in 2007.

Perhaps compounding all of this are changes taking place both in the medical profession and in the pharmaceutical industry. We're heading for an oversupply of doctors – or, as one wag put it, the stream of urologists will dry up, the supply of psychiatrists will shrink, and there'll be cuts among the surgeons. He might have added that it would be rash to predict the future for dermatologists.

The good news is that as the population ages, the amount of money spent on pharmaceuticals goes up, which should act as a stimulant to advertising and promotional spending. Of course, the market is fueled in part by new product launches, and the so-called pipeline for new drugs is rapidly constricting, while patents on existing blockbusters like Claritin expire.

The bad news, at least from the standpoint of medical journal publishers, is that pharmaceutical spending on promoting prescription products direct to consumers now takes up an increasing proportion – close to a quarter, or $3 billion – of the roughly $16 billion a year the industry spends on all forms of marketing.

Moreover, the pharmaceutical companies are no longer allowed to seduce doctors with free dinners. The days of trinkets and junkets are over – by law. Gaining access to physicians in order to discuss drug products is the thing that keeps executives and some 90 000 sales reps awake at night, as I found during a recent research project my company conducted for *Institutional Investor*, a division of Euromoney.

Drug firms will become even more dependent on R&D (they're already spending twice as much as they did a decade ago, and with fewer major new products to show for it) especially with an estimated one-third of the industry's best-selling patents about to expire, and doctors will have to demonstrate, with the help of computers, that their work is cost-efficient. In all of this change, though, I do see a continuing, if different, partnership between the pharmaceutical industry and the medical profession. The industry now has a vested interest in targeted, value-added, informational Continuing Medical Education, and, for that matter, in a sophisticated and discerning consumer.

These developments have a huge impact on medical publishing, which has enjoyed 20 or 30 years of incredible growth connected with developments in research. Yet the explosion of knowledge brought its own problems. Over publication; a cafeteria of choices; a cacophony of messages. Jay Lippincott, CEO of what is now Lippincott, Williams and Wilkins, says the way to get attention amid all of the din is to be market focused, by a redoubled effort at *quality* of content and presentation. Publishers who don't listen to – and respond to – an increasingly discerning and demanding clientele won't survive, he says. And indeed, publishers often think they know what's best for their audience without checking with that audience first. With that in mind, I asked my graduate students at Rosemont to survey doctors about what they read and what they need. Their term project was to produce a publication based upon their findings.

And indeed, publishers have a key role to play in the whole concept of what drug company Eli Lilly calls "knowledge is powerful medicine." But it will be a different role. Those who want to disseminate that knowledge had better be ready for the changes being wrought by volatile advertising support, consumer sophistication, rapid advances in information, and a proliferation of media. The American Medical Publishers Association (AMPA), until quite recently a cozy club of mildly Dickensian *colporteurs,* now has several members who are in purely electronic media.

Part of the tumult in medical publishing – something that a headhunter at last year's AMPA annual meeting called 'not an industry for sissies' – is in the re-shaping of healthcare itself. Specifically, managed care, which is, in effect, healthcare in the US today.

Robert Benchley once observed that the world is divided into two types of people: those who divide the world into two types of people – and those who do not. Where managed care is concerned, there are, it seems, two types – those who hate it; and those who merely loathe it.

Despite studies showing that quality of care has not been demonstrably compromised under managed care, it is hard to find any friends of the system among either doctors or patients. But ask about alternatives, or look for positive articles about managed care and you seek in vain. The media cite horror stories about denial of care; TV series such as *ER* feature doctors trying to do good despite managed care's strictures. And you might remember when audiences applauded loudly when Helen Hunt did an anti-managed care rant a few years ago in the movie *As Good As It Gets*.

All of this, despite the fact that – to paraphrase Winston Churchill on the subject of democracy – managed care is the worst form of healthcare except for all those other forms that have been tried from time to time. I pretty much said this in my Research Report for the *Economist Intelligence Unit* and still have some of the arrows in my back to show for it.

Today, more than 80% of Americans insured by their employers are in some sort of managed care plan – as are the overwhelming majority of doctors.

What does this mean for publishing? I believe it means a whole new set of opportunities. Healthcare professionals are avid for management information, and evidence-based medicine, customer service, and legal and ethical issues are all assuming new significance; new technologies need to be explained; information technology has to be demystified. It's hardly surprising that an estimated 2% of our $1.5 *trillion* a year healthcare system is now spent on consultants trying to figure out, and explain, what's happening!

For medical writers the opportunities are huge. Not only in interpreting the enormous and complex advances in medical science, but also in exploring and clarifying the healthcare delivery issues that affect all of us: affordability is perhaps the main one. But also the need for 'wiring' healthcare; the aging population; increasingly sophisticated (and expensive) technology; malpractice and medical error; consumer power; quality and consistency of care; the 44 million uninsured Americans; the threats posed by biologic, chemical and radiologic weapons; re-thinking the way we train health professionals – viz: narrative medicine – and the continuing, nagging issue of what former Penn professor of medicine Dr Bill Kissick calls "Infinite needs versus finite resources."

Writing in English may be, as James Joyce put it, "the most ingenious torture ever devised for sins committed in previous lives" but the rewards for bringing to bear on medical writing what I call the four Ps – Passion, Perseverance, Patience and Pachydermia (a skin thick enough to deflect criticism) – are enormous.

Moreover, there are international opportunities for medical publishers. Countries in Europe, Asia and Latin America – faced, like the US, with aging populations and ever-more-expensive technology – are looking to American management know-how.

Not that there aren't cultural barriers to global adoption of the managed care model. Other countries don't necessarily share Americans' unique optimism that leads them to believe that, if only they spend enough money on healthcare, death can be postponed – possibly even avoided altogether. As one Scottish physician who moved from Scotland to Canada to California put it: "In Scotland, death is imminent; in Canada, it's inevitable; in California, it's optional."

A quick note on newsletters. The Newsletter Publishers Association has some 700 members representing about 5000 titles of which roughly 300 are on healthcare topics. A study of some 250 newsletter publishers conducted at Northwestern University concluded that: "Though its revenues exceed the billion-dollar level . . . the newsletter industry has been all but ignored by mainstream media and academe. This omission now becomes even more glaring as the [newsletter] industry prepares to go online minus the agony being experienced by many magazine and newspaper companies. The specialty-targeted newsletter seems poised for unprecedented success as it steadily winds its way towards cyber distribution. Already, one-fourth of all for-profit news-letters provide for online delivery." AMPA's own newsletter and *Philadelphia Medicine* – both of which we publish – are available online.

So, with paper costs rising, journal advertising declining, subscription prices forcing libraries – and individuals – to cut back on purchases but still to demand the best and most current information, is the way to do it an electronic way? A superhighway?

Well, radio existed for 38 years before it had 50 million listeners; television took 13 years to reach that number; the Internet got there in just four years. Today, more than two-thirds of US physicians access the Internet . . . with medical libraries and publisher sites ranked highest among doctors who use the web for professional reasons. Even so, some experts warn that although the Internet has provided a way to connect all our computers, training for the use of such technology among medical professionals is lacking. So the use of the Internet to exchange medical information has been sluggish.

Now, I have a confession: My office sports a picture of Johannes Gutenberg, and as one who has thus far failed to extinguish that damn winking sign on my VCR, I am reluctant to claim any special insights about the Internet. In fact, I twice lost chunks of a piece I wrote a couple of years ago for the *Economist Intelligence Unit* on the information highway in healthcare. Furthermore, I take a fugitive pleasure from knowing that two of the most creative science fiction writers and futurists of the 20th century – Isaac Asimov and Ray Bradbury – steadfastly refused to fly in an airplane.

But for those whose knuckles whiten at the mere thought of winging through cyberspace, The Association of American Publishers produced a lucid and balanced document titled *Promises and Pitfalls: a briefing paper on Internet publishing*. It starts with the premise that "Publishers participate in the creation and dissemination of knowledge. We need to remind ourselves as we go along that our ultimate goal is not necessarily the preservation of publishing as we know it. If we – commercial and not-for-profit publishers alike – do not clearly understand this, we will lose our role in the process altogether."

The document lists as advantages: efficiency, decentralized operation, time-liness, searchability, customization, globalization, access and cost. And the disadvantages as: quality control, hidden real costs, copyright, privacy, and a lack of the formal rigor of print. Paul Evan Peters, executive director of the Coalition for Networked Information, likens the present status of the Internet to a "Paleolithic period . . . in which crude tools are being used to fashion crude but functional artifacts; in which the dominant personalities are hunter-gatherers and storytellers; in which institutions and organizations . . . are hard at work securing the gains of these pioneers by constructing fixed settlements that are attractive to settlers."

To be sure, the Internet is more quirky and anarchic – less linear – than print. Whoever said that freedom of the press is greatest for those who own one was unwittingly prescient. Traditional publishing is an *ex cathedra* affair, top-down, hierarchical. Electronic publishing is essentially egalitarian. Not only that, but in the electronic age, publishers may not be the only ones doing the publishing. Universities like USP may be the sleeping giants of publishing, with the World Wide Web having turned every university into a publisher and every faculty member into an author; after all, the university's business is knowledge creation, transmission and management.

And incidentally, anyone who has entered a chat room on the Internet will readily see that it's only a matter of time before we return to grunts and hieroglyphics. In medicine, where clarity and simplicity in communication are vital, there's a crisis. Illegible handwriting is one thing; unintelligible speech and prose are quite another. Physician and author Richard Asher wrote that "to rise quickly in the medical profession you must learn to sell your ideas by acquiring the technique of pseudo-profundity. Remember that the harder anything is to understand," he said, "the more readily will committees allocate money to it. Much sensible medicine is obvious, but the obvious does not impress."

That, I think, is where writers and editors will have their day in the sun: no matter what the medium, language, syntax, cadence, pellucid prose will be more vital – and more in demand – than ever. Any advice for accomplishing all that? Aside for the four Ps – read, read, read. Find a role model such as George Orwell, who in his all-too-brief life (he died of tuberculosis at 47) produced a prolific output of novels and essays.

"Good prose is like a window pane," Orwell wrote in his essay, *Why I Write*. And his attention to clarity of prose is an enduring lesson for those who aspire to express their thoughts clearly. Linguist Geoffrey Nunberg calls Orwell's classic *Politics and the English Language* the most widely-cited of all 20th century essays on the language. In it, Orwell refers to the mixture of vagueness and sheer incompetence that is the most marked characteristic of modern English prose . . . which he says consists less and less of words chosen for their meaning, and more and more of phrases "tacked together like sections of a prefabricated hen house." He warns against worn-out metaphors like having no axe to grind, or mixed metaphors such as the Fascist octopus has sung its swan song.

Above all, Orwell called for sincerity, simplicity, and concreteness in language. The greatest enemy, he believed, is insincerity such as the example he cites in *Politics*: "Defenseless villages are bombed from the air, the inhabitants driven out into the countryside, the cattle machine-gunned, the huts set on fire with incendiary bullets – this is called pacification."

Orwell gives in that essay a wonderful example of linguistic decay. He starts by quoting the well-known verse from *Ecclesiastes*: "I returned and saw under the sun, that the race is not to the swift, nor the battle to the strong, neither yet bread to the wise, nor yet riches to men of understanding, nor yet favor to men of skill; but time and chance happeneth to them all." This he turns into modern English as: "Objective consideration of contemporary phenomena compels the conclusion that success or failure in competitive activities exhibits no tendency to be commensurate with innate capacity, but that a considerable element of the unpredictable must invariably be taken into account."

I would submit, too, that all teaching is firstly the teaching of language. Muddled syntax is the outward and audible sign of confused minds, and the misuse of grammar the result of illogical thinking.

In sum, I see a synergistic broadcasting of information through a variety of media . . . with quality and relevance and credibility of the material being the principal factors governing the user's choice of medium. In fact, the *British Medical Journal* suggests an amalgam of short print articles hitched to a more detailed version of the same thing online. That iconoclastic journal also whimsically leans on *The Simpsons* to illustrate changes in medical publishing.

After noting that such publishing is (quote) changing dramatically because of many forces, the editors posit four possible futures. In the (wise) Marge world, "academics innovate and publish primarily on the web not in journals; publishers must publish large numbers to succeed." In the (lazy) Homer world, "publishers adapt to the electronic world and continue to publish research." In the (well-informed) Lisa world, "publishers have largely disappeared, and communication takes place mainly through global electronic conversations." And in the (street-wise) Bart world, "publishers have largely disappeared, and large organizations have become the main purveyors of research."

As the Association of American Publishers puts it: "There are some who will rightly conclude that the changes (in medical publishing) are so enormous, and that sociological adaptability lags so far behind, that business for print-based publishers will continue to be robust into the 21st century." And *Newsweek* weighs in with a cheery answer to the question: "Will computers kill paper usage?" Not a cyber chance, says the magazine, predicting that the demand for paper for print media will jump from 30 million tons in 1995 to almost 50 million by the year 2015.

But then again, when the telephone came into being, it was predicted that it would bring peace on earth, eliminate accents and class distinctions, revolutionize surgery and stamp out heathenism.

Prediction is an uncertain, yet durable and wonderful business. Perhaps second only to publishing.

David Woods

Physician, heal thyself

Becoming accustomed to public speaking

With the proliferation of medical knowledge and the profusion of seminars and scientific sessions designed to disseminate that knowledge, more and more physicians are being asked to speak in public.

While many of them have mastered the techniques of transmitting information in a winning and influential way, others – regardless of their medical specialty – become effective anesthetists once they get on their feet to speak.

Effective public speakers aren't born, they're made. They're made by practice, complete knowledge of their subject, and the ability to put it across logically, clearly, succinctly, and with evident interest and enthusiasm: monotonous speech – however dramatic its content – will turn listening into listlessness. On the other hand, ringing, Churchillian oratory, while it may have contributed immeasurably to Allied morale in World War Two, carries little weight when used to deliver a paper on acne. In fact, words used for their own sake can, as much in speaking as in writing, serve to obfuscate the omphalos of your subject. Try saying that to an audience at five o'clock in the afternoon.

But there are some guidelines for speakers that will keep verbal genocide on live audiences to a minimum. Speak naturally, clearly, and with the help of notes – and develop your theme logically. A strong start is important since it is vital to show your listeners during the first minute – when you can be sure that you have their attention – that you are not another rambling bore. Then, after developing two or three major points as the core of your discussion, wrap it all up neatly with some clear conclusions: in other words, tell them what you're going to tell them; tell them; then tell them what you've told them. Don't try to pack too much information into your talk; it confuses the audience and does you out of an opportunity to deal with the subject again from another angle – and to accept a further honorarium.

Avoid mannerisms, repetition, and catch phrases. Pruritus ani may be the theme of your talk but scratching yourself there (or anywhere else) will be as irritating and distracting to the audience as it seems to be to the afflicted speaker. Misuse of words, and such excretions as "in solo practice on my own" and "per diem a day," indicate lack of preparation and polish and can annoy even the less pedantic listener. Catch phrases, as one contributor to the *Lancet* noted, can be equally annoying. He referred to a speaker who insisted on introducing illustrations with the comment: "Here's our old friend the giant cell again," and quite properly pointed out that most of the audience were not, and did not intend to be, on friendly terms with a giant cell.

Properly used, however, illustrations do serve to pep up a sagging audience and to refocus attention. They should be relevant, rather than of the home movie variety, of high quality and pictorial. If illustrations are used to present written material, this should be simple and easy to read. The speaker should allow adequate time for their message to sink in, and should avoid showing illustrations with handwritten data or several lines of laborious type that could be better explained verbally. Magnifying the average physician's handwriting so that it's two feet high and in lights is unforgivable and unnecessary.

So, to recap: plan your talk, stick to two or three well-made points, speak from notes or from memory, speak clearly and not too fast – and keep it as short as possible. Be logical, interested, and natural; avoid clichés and mannerisms; use illustrations, jokes, or other devices to keep your audience awake and interested only where these are absolutely relevant.

Answer questions – however silly they may appear to be – with interest, and briefly. Question time isn't an excuse for another full-fledged presentation. Following these guidelines will guarantee you a live audience and, at the end of your talk, a better-informed one. You will have done something to narrow the information gap, and will probably be asked to speak again before long.

Finally, end your speech when you have promised to. The speaker who says "... and in conclusion" more than twice may find that his audience has taken him at his word and gone home.

David Woods

Do you speak "Medispeak"?

Every profession has its jargon, a word that derives from Middle English *gargoun* – twittering of birds. Among insiders, that twittering serves as a specialized and often useful "in" language; even though it's not the vocabulary of everyday speech, it has its place. The problem arises when legalese, journalese, or other forms of jargon are used in communicating with – or in the presence of – outsiders. Then, intentionally or not, it can become exclusionary or threatening. Moreover, where it is meant to impress, or even oppress, it can become a powerful and dangerous weapon.

This is especially true in medicine. While jargon isn't unique to medicine, "Medispeak" – or, as the *Oxford Companion to the English Language* (*OCEL*) dubs it, medicant – certainly isn't new.

The medieval physician Arnold of Villanova suggested that his 13th-century colleagues mask their scientific limitations with lengthy Latinate locutions.

Acknowledging that studies of surgeons have shown that jargon used during surgery actually improved the communication of factual information with clarity and brevity, the *OCEL* goes on to note that "ability to understand and use the jargon of a group is a badge of identification . . . it indicates that the user is conforming to the norms of the group, as well as accepting and understanding [its] basic ideas, principles, and practices."

So, while physicians readily understand that cephalalgia means headache and emesis means vomiting, patients might not; in fact, hearing those words might induce the very conditions they describe. Yet sometimes jargon, when it consists of euphemism or obliqueness, can be a kindness to the patient: better to learn, for instance, that senility is "decreased propensity for cell replication" or that an alcoholic is "suffering from chronic hyperingestion of ethanol."

Of greater concern is the medical "we." Like the royal or the editorial we, it is designed to cloak communication in an aura of respectability and received wisdom, as in "We see a lot of that" or, worse, "How are we today?" The impersonal "emphysema in the corner bed" – the reference to the disease, as opposed to the person with the disease – is in the same place. The same holds true for referring to human beings as cases of this or that. And the "Hi, Mary, I'm Doctor Smith" isn't far behind.

John Gartland MD, author of *Medical Writing and Communicating*, says that the characteristics important to good personal communicating are empathy, trust, honesty, and caring. Physicians, he says, should treat patients as they themselves would want to be treated. He points out that "the use of medical jargon, appearing hurried, or giving patients the sense of begrudging them adequate time to be heard . . . are the most commonly encountered barriers to effective communication between physicians and patients in face-to-face encounters."

The solution to all this? If you think you might be suffering from Medispeak, the humorous answer is to seek out a psychosemanticist who will straighten out any linguistic ailments you might be suffering from. More realistically, speak simply, personally, equitably, and kindly – it's a vital part of the therapeutic process. And you'll probably feel better, too.

David Woods

Let's hear it for sounder listening skills!

"It is the disease of not listening, the malady of not marking, that I am troubled withal," says Sir John Falstaff in *Henry IV*, part two. Sir John's problem isn't new, although Shakespeare's remedy for it – hanging by the heels – was perhaps a bit extreme. In fact, the disease has surely become even more troublesome in recent times, aggravated by our propensity to tune out or switch off entirely the ubiquitous voices of radio and television – and as a result increasingly to do the same to our fellow human beings.

Some of the symptoms of the disease of not listening are impatience, a low threshold for boredom, and irritation when speakers don't provide a "lead paragraph," a clear focal point, or when they engage in the sort of self-indulgent long-windedness that Benjamin Disraeli described as "tracing the steam engine always back to the kettle."

In his book *How to Speak, How to Listen*, Mortimer Adler says that it is utterly amazing how people generally assume that the ability to listen well is a natural gift requiring no training.

"Deficiencies in listening and the ensuing failures in communication," says Adler, "are a major source of wasted time, ineffective operation, and miscarried plans and decisions."

Adler lists some of the bad habits that interfere with proper listening: paying more attention to a speaker's mannerisms while allowing one's mind to wander, overreacting to certain words or phrases that arouse adverse emotional responses, or just daydreaming. Listening, Adler believes, requires penetrating through the words to the thoughts that lie behind them. It calls for sifting what's important from what isn't; it requires perceiving as early as possible the focus of what is being said.

It could be argued that if people spoke more logically and grammatically and colorfully than most of us do, listening would be easier. But that's rather like saying that astronomy would be more rewarding if there were never any clouds.

Philadelphia Inquirer columnist Lona O'Connor lists three types of listening: supportive – making speakers comfortable enough to state what's on their mind; active – asking questions and advancing the conversation; and analytic – figuring out what the information means and what to do about it.

O'Connor adds bluntly: "Can you improve your listening skills? You'd better. Your future could depend on it." This is especially true for healthcare professionals who, by turning an intentionally deaf ear to what's being said or by failing to detect nuance, may place their careers in jeopardy. It's estimated that more than half of all malpractice litigation has its origins in garbled communication and misunderstanding.

So, for improved patient care and decreased risk of litigation, let's hear it for sounder listening. It's an exercise in preventive medicine – and certainly better than the Bard's cure.

David Woods

Specialty scientific meetings: time for critical review

There was a time when theater audiences routinely hurled apple cores or orange peel at actors whose performances they judged to be unworthy. Professional critics have continued the practice using verbal missiles. In her entertaining book, *No Turn Unstoned*, actress Dame Diana Rigg catalogued several of the most deadly of these: "The play opened at 8:40 sharp and closed at 10:20 dull"; "A bad play saved by a bad performance"; and one critic's terse dismissal of *I Am a Camera* – "Me no Leica."

Most medical specialties and subspecialties hold annual or semi-annual scientific meetings and, while the same critical barbs should not necessarily be aimed at their participants, the time has come for honest and stringent appraisal. Such meetings will never improve so long as rambling, inaudible, or boring speakers are accorded the same polite applause as those whose words gladden the ear and stimulate the mind.

There is surely no need for medical meetings where drowsy audiences are forced to succumb to numbing illogic, tortured syntax, and, in many instances, the slings and arrows of outrageous illustrations. Yet people who attend such meetings are a remarkably tolerant and forgiving lot. In the interest of keeping themselves up-to-date with the world of science, they sit in mesmerized silence while their peers recount their scientific triumphs or tell us how to practice more efficiently.

One veteran of the medical meeting wars notes that "we were offered some excellent science, but its impact was seriously impaired by the appalling quality of at least half the presentations." The remark he heard most often was: "Those of you in the back of the room won't be able to see this illustration, but . . ."

Is it asking too much, one wonders, to suggest that skill in communicating with an audience be a prerequisite for membership in the presenters' club?

Those planning specialty meetings can bring some imagination to the task by inquiring of those likely to attend them what subjects they would like to hear about and then matching those subjects with speakers of demonstrated ability.

Didactic presentations, unless about the secrets of the universe, should be limited to 30 minutes. Illustrations should be professionally produced and presented, visible from all areas of the room, and left on the screen long enough to be read.

When the speaker has finished, members of the audience should be encouraged to rate the performance then and there. Beyond such rating, an exercise that in some instances might be the genteel equivalent of throwing apple cores or orange peels, specialty societies might appoint a "meeting critic" who would not only collate the written opinions of the audience, but also write a frank critique in the society's journal of the meeting's content and value – and its high and low moments.

Of course, scientific meetings do not consist only of formal presentations. Many who attend them would agree that their greatest value is to be found in the social areas where exchanges about matters of common professional interest are often more relevant and rewarding. But even these encounters in what used to be called the "smoke-filled rooms" might take on more focus and clarity if there has been some sparkle and fire at the podium, too.

David Woods

Recognizing and avoiding non-verbal cues we give our patients

Ever since the Institute of Medicine's 1999 report suggesting that medical errors represent the eighth-largest cause of death in the US, the medical profession has been scrutinized and criticized, including allegations of ineffectual physician–patient communication. Suggested remedies abound, including a curious law in Washington state requiring physicians to write legibly, the test of their legibility being whether involved nurses or pharmacists can read their writing. A successful professional response to these criticisms must begin by each individual doctor remembering that treating disease and caring for patients are not necessarily the same activity.

Experts say that between 55% and 70% of physician–patient communication is non-verbal. Only about 7% comprises actual words used, the rest consisting of physician tone of voice, physician posture, physician facial expressions, and physician actions suggesting to patients the interaction will soon be over.

National surveys show that 21% of native-born adults cannot read a newspaper front page, and 48% cannot read a timetable. How, then, can we expect all patients to understand written follow-up or discharge instructions, or to read medication labels? Also, many patients are less than conversant in English and fail to grasp what we are telling them.

Resolving these situations requires more of the art of medicine than of the science of medicine. We can improve both our patient care and our professional image by being more aware of the need to address not only the biological but also the psychological, social, and cultural factors that accompany illness in our patients.

This means:

- recognizing, and avoiding, negative non-verbal clues given to our patients
- making certain patients understand both physician and medication instructions, even if it means using a translator
- treating patients as human beings rather than viewing them as sick bodies
- caring for the whole patient while treating the patient's illness
- curing sometimes, relieving often, and comforting always
- performing like the good doctors we are.

John Gartland MD

Strategies for not appearing rushed

One of the most critical elements in creating the right environment for patients entering your office is the initial 30 seconds. Too often this period is neglected, and practices miss a golden opportunity to begin that relationship on a good note. It may be that the importance of the initial greeting is undervalued because the receptionist is on the phone, tending to a patient, or busy doing paperwork during this interval.

A receptionist's primary responsibility is to greet that patient as he or she comes through the door and thus set the entire tone for the relationship.

This task of greeting patients is not a matter of "time," it is a matter of "tone." It does not take more than five or ten seconds, and certainly in total not more than 30 seconds to greet patients with a warm "Hello" and make them feel welcome and secure. If you are able to accomplish this, not only will you have set the right tone, but the wait in the reception area will be easier. The patients who feel they are nothing more than another number can cause the disconnect responsible for most professional liability lawsuits and poor patient satisfaction ratings.

The quality of the exchange between physician and patient – in other words, the tone – can be helped by such strategies as sitting down to talk to a patient instead of standing above, not looking at your watch, asking open-ended questions, and not interrupting. All this can help you to appear unhurried.

The same is true of explaining and talking about a surgical procedure or a treatment regimen. Giving patients time to ask questions at the end of the visit or when scheduling takes place leaves an impression, either positive or negative, depending on the tone of that interaction.

These communication skills are important for both doctor and staff. Once learned, they are habit forming and will simply begin to become part of the culture of your practice.

James Saxton

Doctors can deliver hope as well as facts of prognosis

Your patient is a 45-year-old professional man with no previous medical history. A lump in his neck caused his internist to refer him to you, an oncologist. The pathology report states that he has anaplastic thyroid cancer (ATC).

It is one of the rarest, deadliest forms of an extremely uncommon cancer. Much of the literature points to a grim prognosis, with a median survival of two years. Most doctors recommend chemotherapy and radiation, but the cancer usually returns. Still, except for the lump in his neck, he appears healthy – and hopeful.

What do you tell him?

If you're like many physicians, you repeat the above prognosis almost verbatim. Many doctors, not wanting to give false hope, offer a basic bottom line of months or years. But this approach often doesn't take into account other variables.

For instance, many might not tell the patient that the fact that he is 20 years younger than the average ATC patient, and that he is in otherwise good health, bodes well for him. Many also might omit the fact that a median survival of two years means only that the middle person in a particular trial – say, the 11th person in a 21-person study – lived two years, but others lived longer, possibly much longer. They would simply say: "Mr Patient, your prognosis is grim. According to the studies, the median survival is two years. I recommend radiation and chemotherapy, but the cancer will probably return." Still others would advise the patient to get his affairs in order and enjoy what time remains.

Do these doctors help their patients by telling this truth? Not necessarily. Although this part of the message is important, there is another element that should not be overlooked.

Because, according to Bernie Siegel MD, who wrote *Love, Medicine and Miracles* and other books on this subject, individuals are not statistics, and there are many people walking around today who, according to medical data, should be dead. And, as many others point out, a patient's mental state dictates, in large part, the progress of his disease. If your patient is frightened or defeated by the truth he or she hears, chances for survival may take a nosedive.

The patient described above is my friend. His doctors recited, almost verbatim, the prognosis in the first paragraph. When he called me, he was considering suicide, rather than face such a painful, ugly death.

I went online. There, I found the doctor's version of the truth. The words "grim prognosis" cropped up liberally in the medical literature. But I also found more. A few patients have lived over five years with no recurrence. One 1995 study said two ATC patients survived over 10 years. This patient's fiancée, who happens to be my sister, found that a doctor she knows had a patient who is a 25-year survivor of ATC. Then I discovered that a recent phase I clinical trial using a new anti-angiogenesis drug led to a (so far) complete three-year remission in one ATC patient. I tracked down this survivor, who led me to his doctor. Although my friend didn't qualify for this particular clinical trial, further research led to an oncologist with a special interest in anti-angiogenesis, who agreed to treat him.

What is the truth of his situation now? Most important, it has changed drastically from one of wait-and-die to proactivity – with hope, and the possibility of a positive outcome.

In my years as a patient mentor, I have been puzzled by doctors who feel that giving patients false hope is wrong. Hope alone has kept many patients alive for years beyond their expected survival time.

So how can you tell the truth in a way that will help your patients?

- Never speak in totally negative terms. Remember, no truth is ever simple. There are always people who survive even the deadliest forms of every disease. It also can be helpful to double-check the latest research before talking with a patient with a troubling diagnosis. In this scientific age, new treatments are discovered daily.
- Encourage patients to research their conditions. Although this may be more time-consuming for you, your patients will enjoy working with you and may have better outcomes.
- Don't discourage your patients from trying so-called unproven remedies. Instead, help them choose those with the most promise – in addition to the traditional treatments you recommend. Many mainstream medical establishments, including academic and research institutions, already have begun to move in this direction.
- Encourage your patients to research nutritional solutions. More and more, the role of nutrition is being viewed as integral both to the prevention and treatment of even the most life-threatening diseases.
- Don't forget how important your attitude is to your patients' survival. Most patients regard their doctors as authorities – "If my doctor said it, it must be true." So be careful what you say. A tone of pessimism can negatively influence your patients' outcomes. Similarly, your positive attitude can lead to better outcomes.

Here are two stories, both about neurosurgeons at a Midwestern medical center. Both patients had cancerous brain tumors.

The first neurosurgeon told his patient about the severity of his condition, adding that the median survival is one year. When the patient asked if he had a chance, the doctor raised his eyes, looked heavenward and said sadly, "I could win the lottery, too." This patient died within months.

The second neurosurgeon gave his patient the same information, but omitted the median survival time. He ended by cheerfully putting his arm around his patient and saying: "But I think we're going to do just fine!"

These words, spoken 10 years ago, echo in my mind today. This doctor was my husband's neurosurgeon and my husband is still alive – eight years after the literature would have predicted his death.

I am not discounting my husband's determination and grit; nor am I discounting the wonders of modern surgery and pharmacology; or my own devotion and nutritional, home-cooked meals. But I am thankful that our neurosurgeon believed that there is no such thing as false hope. This approach can serve as a reminder for others of the healing power and potential of the physician's own words.

Julia E Schopick

The doctor patient

Aside from physicians having a lower incidence of arteriosclerotic disease and a higher one of suicide, their causes of death aren't much different from those of the general population, according to a study of more than 1200 physicians' deaths in five American states. Moreover, studies by the American Medical Association show that physicians have a life expectancy that is two to three years longer than that of their same-aged, non-physician counterparts.

These statistics might seem strange in light of the litany of lethal stresses allegedly afflicting the medical profession. These have been documented variously as the emotional battering of being confronted with the daily prospect and often actuality of pain and death, time pressures, the threat of malpractice suits, decreased autonomy, increased regulation, increased competition from newly minted physicians and allied healthcare workers, and the difficulties the helping professions have in measuring accomplishment.

An Australian study concluded that "when doctors need doctors they are even worse off than lawyers who need lawyers, for law only involves a sapiential authority while medicine is concerned with the less well defined, elusive, yet more pervasive medical authority." In fact, a study comparing the ways in which physicians and lawyers handle stress found that lawyers tolerate frustration and tiredness better than physicians and that lawyers take more time off to relax. The study concluded that "all other professional stresses are resisted better by lawyers and stressors are fewer. Drinking habits in response to stress are identical . . . [and] the rate of divorce is approximately equal."

So as far as dealing with their own stress and disease is concerned, physicians suffer from what the Australian study describes as "therapeutic nihilism," deferring attention to serious symptoms and being the worst conformers to a schedule of therapeutic administration. The study concludes not with "Physician, heal thyself," but "Physician, know thyself." Explore your limitations and without humility acknowledge your strengths, and talk out the problem and open up perspectives to family and close friends.

In a Louis Harris poll of 1430 practitioners, 50% of whom said that they would not recommend medicine as a career as highly as they would have ten years earlier, loss of autonomy, loss of personal satisfaction, and excessive personal demands were the principal reasons cited. One prescription for physicians who are burned out or discontented: reverse the work obsession; allow yourself to enjoy your job; redefine "yourself" from within, independently of your profession; commit yourself to personal health; and take responsibility for your own happiness. All of which may not improve the life expectancy of physicians but could go a long way toward improving their lives.

David Woods

The importance of doctors' "people skills"

"My doctor doesn't talk to me" and "My doctor doesn't tell me anything about my condition" are complaints frequently voiced by patients. Good relationships between doctors and patients have long been recognized as a critical alliance by the medical profession, but seem to be honored more frequently in the breach than in the attainment by some doctors. A belief persists that interpersonal problems arising between doctors and patients are aggravated by the sense that some doctors emphasize curing over caring.

Too often doctors regard the art of medicine, bedside manner, and "people skills" with suspicion because the scientific basis for these interpersonal interactions seems to lack the objectivity of René Laennec, the 18th-century French physician credited with inventing the stethoscope, who reputedly advised his nephew that, even though doctors might think it silly, doctors hold their credit solely from the public and it would be foolish for young doctors not to respect this role of the public.

Medical practice must become more socially conscious and responsive to the needs of its patients. This calls for a shift from a paternalistic "doctor knows best" type of medical practice to a more egalitarian model characterized by the consent process and shared decision making. Knowing what is best for patients remains an acceptable reason for doctors to act on their behalf, provided patients are fully informed of the reasons for the actions and are offered the opportunity to be part of the decision-making process.

Some hospitals and health centers are beginning to ask their patients to rate their doctors' communication skill and availability, as well as the technical aspects of the care received. This becomes a new and compelling reason for doctors to take stock of their patient communication and interpersonal skills.

Some institutions may include provisions for added reimbursements or bonuses tied to performance targets set by the organization. Incentive bonus plans offered to participating doctors by these organizations are usually tied to scores obtained by rating doctors on patient satisfaction, quality of care, and cost-effectiveness. Doctors who consistently receive low scores on these imposed criteria not only may be denied bonus payments but also could lose patients. This is certainly sufficient motivation to be certain you have good "people skills."

John Gartland MD

The profession's image: you're OK, they're not

The story of the foreign resident in the US who, having enquired about his patient's health, and on being told, "Gee, Doc, I feel lousy" began to examine the patient's scalp in search of pediculus capitis, may well be apocryphal. It would be nice if the question of the medical profession's current image could be dealt with in such a blissful manner.

You don't think the medical profession's image is lousy? Well, in a literal sense, it's probably no more so than the resident's patient, but through accumulated misunderstanding and poor communication it's come to look that way. The fact is that most people are very fond of "my" doctor, but when they're asked to give their views on the medical profession as a whole – made up, as it is, of "my" doctors – the attitude becomes quite different.

This strange public projection that one physician is okay, but physicians *en masse* are not to be trusted at any cost, is unfortunately perpetuated by doctors themselves; instead of viewing it, as their training equips them to do, as an interesting socio-medical problem, they go on the defensive.

How has this arisen? Well, it's been said that patients are physically, mentally, and morally naked when being examined by doctors, and if this is true it can hardly be considered conducive to a comfortable relationship. But this isn't really the problem. The trouble stems from the time, not too long ago, when apotheosizing the physician became unfashionable and stopped; when patients ceased to marvel, as listeners to Oliver Goldsmith's village parson did, "that one small head could carry all he knew." Awe of the physician gave way to grudging acceptance; gratitude grew into demand. Not only that but physicians are often unwillingly cocooned by sycophants – employees who manage to give the public an impression of medical practice quite different from that which the doctor would want to project. Receptionists and other employees, for example, can sometimes be brusque and unhelpful to patients, seeing themselves as custodians of the medical practice and defenders of its practitioners.

Medicine has been described as the only profession that labors incessantly to destroy the reason for its own existence. But that's no reason why the great majority of its practitioners should masochistically allow themselves to be burned at the stake of public awareness. It's time doctors made the public aware that they spend six to ten or more years learning their trade; that a union plumber who put in a 60- or 70-hour-work week would likely earn more money than they do; that overheads can swallow up to 30–50% of their gross income; that they can't be held responsible for all of society's ills; that they can treat, for instance, the effects of poverty but that they cannot single-handedly eliminate the disease of poverty itself.

Let's get some public acknowledgement that 99 out of 100 physicians are doing a conscientious and dedicated job. Before the current wave of medicophobia becomes irreversible there must be a concerted effort to make the public aware of this.

How to do it? It would be easy to say bring on the image makers to patch up the profession's public perception. Don't apologize for the fact that you earn X thousand a year when your training, long hours, and the importance of what you're doing merit above average financial reward. Don't apologize for the fact that you're not, white knight-wise, putting a stop to pollution, racial inequality, or war. On the other hand, instead of meeting criticism of incompetence with the mumbled "few rotten apples in every basket," encourage public knowledge about the delivery of health services. Moreover, rather than taking a defensive attitude towards healthcare, physicians are ideally placed to educate: to be more active and vociferous. They can, for instance, liaise with the politicians in shaping future health services, and they can work in the schools in an effort to shape future health practices.

And your best weapon in improving communication with the public is the plain truth. If you think you're doing a good job and a vital one – say so.

David Woods

What's wrong with a little "loathsome finery"?

In his book *Harley Street*, Reginald Pound wrote that "a motor car was advertised for sale in the early 1920s as 'especially built to suit the wearer of a top hat in comfort and therefore admirably adapted to the needs of a Harley Street specialist'." Pound added that while the war banished the silk hat as a sartorial "must" for fashionable London physicians, "some consultants were reluctant to shed what Hazlitt called 'the loathsome finery of the profession of blood'."

But the notion of a distinctive – albeit more utilitarian – uniform for physicians persists in the form of the white coat. And patients seem to like it. A study of 200 patients at two teaching hospitals found that more than half preferred their doctors to wear white coats, a finding that prompted the researchers who conducted the study to conclude that "the white coat remains a powerful symbol" and that "physicians should adopt formal standards in attire as well as speech to avoid alienating . . . patients."

White, supposedly, is the color of power – and not merely for coats. It is the most popular color for such automobile status symbols as Jaguar and Mercedes. And even though Samuel Johnson observed that "fine clothes are good only as they supply the want of other means of procuring respect," clearly a white-coated physician is more credible than one wearing, say, jeans and a t-shirt.

The physician's credibility may rest as much on address as dress. A *Journal of the American Medical Association* article cites the "Hi, Mary, this is Dr Smith" exchange as a particularly unfortunate juxtaposition of the informal and the formal that can turn a patient apoplectic. The way the exchange should go is "Hi, Mary, this is Jim" or "Hi, Ms Jones, this is Dr Smith."

Says physician–author Lester S King: "Asymmetrical address between doctor and patient encourages condescension in personal relationships . . . If you are a mature patient and your doctor calls you by your first name, then in return address him by his first name." On balance, though, the white coat may not be all that loathsome and the ms– or mister–doctor exchange might work best; after all, the physician–patient relationship is not a social one.

David Woods

Physicians: an endangered species?

Present manpower data, inconclusive as they are, don't exactly suggest that physicians are an endangered species, although in some rural areas of the country extinction is a real threat. But in a more literal sense doctors are in danger. It's not the perceived danger of a bad press or of being enmeshed in the mad machinery of bureaucracy – it's the very real threat of violence from patients.

Physicians might regard such an occupational hazard as a remote one – about as likely as being struck by lightning or sustaining injury while playing chess – but some medical associations have already drawn up a list of registered dangerous patients, and others are planning to do so.

Medicine, as the *British Medical Journal* has noted, is a high-risk profession; in an age of declining manners, enhanced expectations and, often, impatience for instant gratification, it is getting even more hazardous. The threat is not only from paranoid schizophrenics or patients with dementia, who may become physically or verbally aggressive: it is also from abusers of such drugs as amphetamines, barbiturates, and even cocaine, who may be tempted to abuse doctors in order to get more of those drugs.

Lists of dangerous patients may be one solution; but physicians can't be protected by scraps of paper. While there is no guerilla manual for doctors, one precaution might be a discreetly hidden alarm bell to summon help. Playing it cool and avoiding sudden movements that might be interpreted as threatening are also helpful. There are no posthumous awards for gallantry in such cases.

Psychiatrists and, to a lesser extent, family physicians are especially vulnerable. One psychiatrist attributes the growing danger to a tendency of law enforcement people to refer psychopaths and others to medicine, and to define as mental illness what used to be plain badness. He also believes that the authority of professionals has declined greatly over the last decade or two, and that this begins in the schools: "Twenty years ago," he says, "kids couldn't get away with bad behaviour; now they can. They view professional people as servants of the community who can be maltreated with impunity."

Overall, the matter merits more research. Practically nothing has been written about it. For the moment it is something that calls for vigilance, judgment, common sense, and attention to the laws of probability – attitudes that would have saved von Gudden, physician to mad King Ludwig of Bavaria, who unwisely went for a walk alone with the monarch and was drowned by him.

David Woods

Manners and medicine

The Romans regarded medicine as an inferior occupation, and in Western societies until well into the 18th century the patient dominated the relationship with the physician. Then as medicine became more scientific and complex its practitioners came to be viewed with respect and even awe.

Today, in an age of egalitarianism and consumerism, the doctor–patient relationship appears to be at a stand-off. To some extent this is brought about by the intrusion of more and more technology and its tendency to depersonalize the relationship; the breakdown leads to non-compliance, doctor shopping, and increasing litigation.

What's been lost in all of this is manners. One cannot be genuinely courteous without having regard for the feelings and general welfare of one's fellows – and that applies as much to the patient as to the physician.

The parents of a 15-year-old boy who had spent a couple of weeks in an intensive care unit and received superb medical and nursing care noted that courteous, sensitive communication was in short supply. The boy, having suffered a cerebral vascular accident, was "out of it." Yet when he uttered a fairly mild expletive the nurse castigated his "crudeness." Even when he became more alert, teams of residents grouped themselves around his bed with serious faces and with references to him in the third person, including references to his somewhat poor prognosis at the time.

In such circumstances regressive behavior is to be expected. Hospital workers should be satisfied with whining, demanding patients who are probably getting better care than the silent ones. Many hospital routines can easily be modified to reflect more concern for the patient's physical comfort and mental security.

Norman Cousins, a former editor of *Saturday Review* and author of *Anatomy of an Illness*, who taught literature and communication to medical students at the University of California at Los Angeles, put it well in *The Physician In Literature*. He said: "The responsible physician is more than just a scientist able to make a difficult diagnosis; he is a human being whose skill depends as much on his knowledge of life as it does on his knowledge of disease. Proper treatment calls for an awareness of human uniqueness and for sensitivity to all the elements of human potentiality. Poetry cannot replace prescriptions but it can widen perceptions. What we learn from the world's great literature is that the best education for the physician is a blend of science and the liberal arts."

Not that a knowledge of literature itself leads to good manners. In fact, Dr Samuel Johnson once said that politeness is fictitious benevolence. But surely an understanding of the human condition leads to a greater sensitivity in treating it.

David Woods

Improving physicians' grades in communication

Criticizing physicians is a popular trend, but one frequently cited fault that seems to have substance is the patient complaint that doctors are unwilling to listen to them or to talk with them about their health problems.

The San Francisco-based Pacific Business Group on Health published a study of patient satisfaction with medical groups and physician networks in California and the Pacific Northwest. Results were based on responses from 31 000 patients at 58 voluntarily participating groups. "Overall satisfaction with doctor" gained a 79% rating, but "interpersonal communication" gained only a 65% rating. If doctors score a 65 on a medical school test, they fail the course.

This failing grade on interpersonal communication should act as an alarm bell. Listening and communicating are ancient therapeutic arts that should not be sacrificed to the severe strains associated with rapid changes in the economics of medical practice. Listening to and communicating with patients is an essential part of good patient care, but many patients believe that doctors don't do it well. Physicians like to believe they deliver good patient care in a competent and compassionate manner, but they may be deluding themselves if this care is not accompanied by listening to and communicating with the patient.

The physician–poet William Carlos Williams spoke of this failing when he wrote: "Do we not see that we are inarticulate? That is what defeats us. It is our inability to communicate to another how we are locked within ourselves, unable to say the simplest thing of importance to one another . . . that gives the physician his opportunity."

We won't get a passing grade on interpersonal communication until we improve the quality of our interpersonal exchanges by listening to and communicating well with our patients.

John Gartland MD

How to avoid getting kicked by the media donkey

Being prepared for the media interview will save physicians from embarrassment and reverberation after the fact.

After losing the election for governor of California, Richard Nixon told members of the press that they "wouldn't have Nixon to kick around anymore." Well, as we know, they did. But physicians can avoid being kicked by the media donkey if they understand this creature and learn how to treat it with firmness and respect.

First of all, remember that the donkey thinks it's a thoroughbred racehorse and wants everyone to admire it for its fine breeding, configuration, and form. The media want to attract the attention of readers, listeners, and advertisers. Understanding that will help you get through the interview process unscathed.

Increasingly, reporters from the ranks of both print and electronic journalism are seeking out physicians to comment on aspects of healthcare, both clinical and, more often these days, socio-political. How to remain unscathed – or unkicked?

- Be prepared. Nothing causes readers to turn the page or listeners and viewers to switch stations more than dry, rambling responses. You are, after all, the expert. But being the expert isn't enough. Attention spans are contracting while sources of information are expanding, so you should have a very clear idea – in advance of the interview – of the message you want to convey.
- Be wary. Ill-considered, off-the-cuff remarks can be ruinous. Keep in mind the absolute finality of the printed or broadcast word. Don't be like the physician who mused, on air, about the desirability of sterilizing all welfare mothers with two or more children. He lived to regret the comment for the rest of his rather foreshortened career in medical politics.
- Wariness should extend to realizing that the donkey doesn't only kick defensively; it may do so pre-emptively – even capriciously. *Time* magazine, in its earlier incarnations, would describe an interviewee it didn't like as, say, "portly and aging."
- Be clear. Remember that the educational levels of those to whom your message is beamed differ – unless you're being interviewed in a scientific journal. So, no polysyllabic words, arcane references, or medical jargon.
- Be patient. Interviewers serve as intermediaries between the expert and the audience; they need your help and understanding in order to interpret and present facts.
- Be humble. If you don't know the answer, admit it. Far better to acknowledge ignorance cheerfully and openly than to prove it by hedging and waffling.
- Be cool. Aggressive interviewers, or those with particular axes to grind, should not be allowed to wear you down; nor should those who pose the same question in several different ways. Say something like "A more useful question might be X" rather than "That's a really silly question."

To avoid the media donkey's kick, understand the creature, be firm, make your intent clear, be confident but wary – and humble enough to know that it is bigger than you.

David Woods

Reading to keep up to date

Trying to keep up with medicine's Brobdingnagian strides becomes, almost daily it seems, an apparently impossible task; a task so formidable that many of us might just stop trying. Like George Orwell's proletarians, 90% of the population might eventually prefer to remain in a permanent state of befuddlement on Victory gin while being ruled by an élite minority of omniscient masters. But it is possible to take a more optimistic view of the physician's ability and willingness to absorb information by reading.

This optimism may be well-founded: book publishers show no evidence of being about to leap in despair from high places; general and professional magazines are for the most part thriving. But time is a real problem in trying to plan a reading program. The average adult spends 52 minutes a day reading; and this figure apparently includes all forms of reading from the morning cornflakes packet to the evening newspaper and the bedtime novel.

But the average adult doesn't work a 60-hour week, nor is he in a position where failure to keep up with advances in his professional field could have such far-reaching consequences. Much of the physician's reading has to be done on the run, or during gaps in the line-ups of patients.

Are there means by which the busy physician can keep up by reading? Well, speed-reading may be one solution but this is rather like bolting a good meal in five minutes – probably just as much nourishment, but not very enjoyable. In any case, it's not the mindless devouring of words that counts so much as remembering what you have read. Perhaps a better approach, if a systematic reading program is going to be more than a chore, is to presort the mountain of reading material that may be threatening to avalanche your desk, and turn it into a manageable molehill. One way of doing this is to make full use of abstracts and contents pages in the medical journals, or to circle promising headlines. No paper or magazine can expect to print material that will involve all of its readers all of the time, but nearly all of them make it as easy as possible for readers to pick out what information they need. Just as the executive, to remain effective, has to use time wisely and juggle priorities appropriately, those who want to be informed should try to decide in advance what they want to be informed about and where they can find that information. A process, in other words, of discernment and discipline.

Discipline in reading consists of allotting realistic amounts of time to it; discernment in sifting information; in knowing what not to read. Or, as one writer puts it: "The art of reading is to skip judiciously."

For a month's reading that might include a dozen or more medical journals, several general magazines, and perhaps five or six books, plan ahead, noting those items that will be of interest, and unashamedly leaning on the comments and suggestions of book reviewers with established credibility.

After that, reading becomes constant assessment: is the message coming through? Is the material interesting? Is it enjoyable? These are factors that are not always easy to discern since education, which taught us how to read, has not always taught us how to judge what is worth reading and persevering with.

David Woods

Are postgraduate courses necessary?

Are postgraduate courses any use? Like the curate's egg, they're probably good in parts. Certainly, no one would quarrel with their objectives of keeping physicians up to date and improving patient care. But do they achieve these goals? And do they keep physicians up to date enough – and improve patient care measurably?

If they do fulfill these purposes they probably do so only indirectly. For instance, the therapy for physicians who go to such courses and meetings must be tremendous: safely checked in to a large hotel, and preferably unreachable by electronic means, they are insulated from the demands of patients and able to spend time with their colleagues. When they return to practice, they'll feel better – and patient care will presumably improve in some measure. But meanwhile what have physicians learned in the scientific sessions that they will (a) remember and (b) use?

Quite possibly, all that's needed is some market research into what kinds of postgraduate courses work. It's no use, for example, providing an unsuspecting audience with a lengthy lecture on plantar warts just because someone on the organizing committee knows Fred so-and-so who will speak interminably on that subject at the drop of a hat. And once it's clearly established what people would like to learn about – let's give it to them. Audiences should then be asked afterwards what they liked, and what they learned, so that future courses can be planned accordingly.

Perhaps, too, in planning postgraduate courses we should get away from the idea that the doctor is always the captive audience to be talked at. Let's have more experience-sharing talks from doctors; at least the practitioner doing the talking would learn something, even if nobody else did. Another aid to postgraduate courses: readable illustrations. Putting the equivalent of three journal pages on a screen and flipping to the next graphic in 30 seconds obviously won't teach anybody very much.

After market research, postgraduate courses could do with something else – an element of fun. There's an earnestness about most of them; a feeling that the learning part is something to be got over as quickly as possible.

The thing to aim for is more participatory learning; more debate and discussion. In that way, perhaps postgraduate courses can become more useful and stimulating by turning audiences into active participants rather than passive listeners.

David Woods

Doctor-to-doctor communication

Most professional communications between doctors are in writing, and usually involve consultations, referrals, patient medical records, or published medical articles. But these communications can fail to achieve their purpose because of careless writing, poor word choice, or confusing sentence structure, thus defeating both the purpose and the meaning of the written materials.

Investigators at Nottingham University in the UK studied the quality and education content of communications between consulting orthopedic surgeons and referring general practitioners.

They found that questions asked in the referral letters were rarely answered in the consultants' replies. This negative finding was caused either by the poor writing skill of the practitioners or by the consultants ignoring the stated requests for patient education expressed in the referral letters. Such communication breakdowns tell us that doctors' written materials should be composed in a simple, spare style, should pose or answer questions clearly, should be grammatically correct, and should be constructed in logically derived written sequences.

Physicians frequently ask other physicians to consult on a patient under their care. Both the referring and the consulting physicians have an obligation to the patient, and to each other, to ensure that the consultation is carried out expeditiously, and that breakdowns in the referral or consultation process do not occur.

Both referring and consulting physicians must make certain that all parties involved in the consultation process are adequately informed, both initially and on a continuing basis, during the interaction. As important and necessary as consultations are for providing good medical care, poorly managed consultations can be a source of frustration and anger for patients, patients' families, and involved physicians.

Since a frequent cause of poorly managed consultations is inadequate communication between referring and consulting physicians, doctors should attach to doctor-to-doctor communications the same degree of importance they attach to physician–patient relationships.

John Gartland MD

Controlling the information balloon

The term "information explosion" has long been consigned to the ranks of cliché. Yet, for medicine, the problem it defined is still very much with us. According to the *British Medical Journal* (*BMJ*) there are over 20 000 biomedical journals – roughly twice as many as 15 years ago.

This sort of exponential growth (there were only 4000 such journals 30 years ago) is not so much an explosion – an expansion with force and noise – as a relentless swelling and distension: an information balloon. Whether this balloon can withstand continued inflation or will be burst by seemingly more streamlined conveyances, such as electronic communication, remains to be seen. But many of the new medical journals coming on the scene, at the rate of 6% to 7% a year, do so, according to the *BMJ*, "because existing ones overlook the fact that the disciplines of many readers cross rigid boundaries – for instance, there are not pure cardiologists but chemical pathologists or immunologists with an interest in cardiology."

This crossover factor is something the American Medical Association (AMA) has referred to as the hidden health system. The AMA has unearthed a growing tendency for physicians in dozens of specialties to provide a significant volume of patient care that is not focused on their particular area of expertise. Thus, many family physicians (FPs) are beginning to specialize in dermatology, and gynecology in primary care. This is reflected in the fact that AMA members, who receive as a perquisite of membership the *Journal of the American Medical Association* and one of nine specialty publications of their choice, are showing an increasing eclecticism: FPs will choose journals on internal medicine, psychiatrists those on neurology, and so on.

So, one way to control the information balloon is to provide in medical journals high-quality scientific articles that cater to a heterogeneous "crossover" readership. If, given that doctors allegedly spend an average of 12.3 hours a month reading professional journals, one can hitch the scientific content to information on medical politics, economics, and practice management, so much the better. After all, physicians are not merely sponges to absorb knowledge – they are human beings with a desire to be educated and informed, and even entertained, in a civilized manner.

It is quality, utility, and versatility that will serve, in the end, to stop the information balloon from bursting.

David Woods

Managing your practice

How your staff can make or break your practice

In airline talk, getting there is supposed to be half the fun. In the practice of medicine, getting patients into the doctor's office is all too often a pretty unhappy journey. But it doesn't have to be. The patient comes to your office to see you – a mutually beneficial meeting, one hopes, that can be arranged with a minimum of fuss.

Trouble is, the poor patient may have to negotiate a number of roadblocks along the way – obstacles of which the physician may be quite unaware. Among these may be a surly and impersonal telephone answering service, an undertrained or overprotective staff, a botched appointments system or that commonest of ailments, excessively cooled heels from undue delay in the waiting room.

Obviously, in a busy office practice a certain amount of turbulence and delay are bound to occur. But a sensitive staff can see to it that these are kept to a minimum.

Let's take a look first at that often blunt instrument, the telephone. Generally, the patient's first step on the journey to your office is to phone for an appointment. Outside office hours the patient will probably encounter the answering service, and this can be a chilling experience.

You may feel that the answering service is beyond your jurisdiction; but, to your patients, its voice might just as well be your own. Say when you'll be back in the office or where you can be contacted in an emergency or who's standing in for you.

So much for matter. When it comes to manner, the answering service may be more difficult. But you can spot-check once in a while. If you encounter one of those bored, hollow voices that manage to convey the impression that something far more critical has been interrupted, make sure that the answering service knows that you expect a better reception for your patient and better value for your money.

Closer to home, telephone communication from your own office will likely be the biggest single factor – after yourself – on which your practice is judged. This is one area where your staff can make or break you – the latter perhaps unwittingly as a result of well-meant attempts to protect the physician from a variety of real or imagined evils: overwork, trivia, etc. In many offices the person responsible for handling the telephone assumes a proprietary protectiveness over the physician, managing to convey the impression that all would be fine in the office were it not for all those bothersome patients.

The solution is to hire a receptionist or secretary who can bring warmth, interest, briskness, judgment, and initiative to the telephone – someone who will smooth the patient's journey to your office, rather than obstruct it. And that, really, is the major part of the answer to all of your staff problems – choosing the right people to work with you in the first place. You wouldn't, after all, select a professional partner with whom you enjoyed no compatibility, or whose working competence you doubted. Why then use anything less than the highest standards to bring in ancillary staff whose impact on your practice may be just as great?

The time to tell all (and to ask all) is at the interview with a prospective employee. Describe in detail the precise nature of the job, the hours, pay, fringe benefits, vacation arrangements; for the successful applicant all of this might profitably be written into a formal contract. In return, you should enquire about experience, references, skills, interests, and career goals, while attempting to discern the applicant's personal suitability to fit in with existing staff and deal pleasantly and intelligently with patients.

Hiring the right person for the right job doesn't mean that you can sit back and consider yourself an Enlightened Employer. Once you've found good people to work with you, keeping them is largely a matter of effective communication.

The first step toward achieving that is for you, the boss, to make your employees aware that they are a vital part of your practice. That doesn't mean just giving them an occasional pat on the head; rather, it ought to involve immediate appreciation for a job well done, or for extra service such as unscheduled overtime.

Two-way communication might also be organized on a regular, structured basis: weekly or monthly staff meetings are a good idea. They can be used not only to discuss the workings of the practice but also to air personal views related to the job. Knowing how to do the job is, as we've seen, mainly a matter of experience. But jobs change as new knowledge and techniques become available.

Today, it's more important than ever that physicians get good value out of their office staff. That's not to suggest slave-driving tactics, but rather a careful look at who's doing what – and how well. Is there duplication of effort? Is there underemployment of some staff members, inappropriate employment of others?

However, it shouldn't take four years of business school to bring about a good working relationship with your office staff. The application of common sense and interpersonal skills ought to be enough, and most doctors have enough of both to make up for a notoriously haphazard medical school training in management techniques.

David Woods

Improving your efficiency by maximizing your time

Organization is not an option; it is mandatory. Start by organizing your administrative staff and business office. Review your charts. They should be organized in a consistent manner that makes it easy to retrieve information. All charts should be pulled in advance of patient appointments and should include appropriate billing forms.

Teach your office staff how to sort mail to improve efficiency. Make sure they understand that mail marked "confidential" is not to be opened by anyone but you. Have other mail sorted in order of priority. Review both correspondence from referring physicians and test results daily. Have your staff put your magazines and journals in one pile and all other non-essential mail in another pile. Make sure your office has a space where you can return charts and other documents to be filed; filing should be done each day.

Next, tackle your office. Plan to spend a Saturday or Sunday clearing your personal work space. Your goal is to remove all non-essential articles and papers from your desk. Create several "in" bins. The first bin should contain only your daily essentials or priority mail, such as referring physicians' letters and test results (attached to the appropriate charts), as well as any other documents requiring your immediate attention. Make sure nothing else creeps into this bin, which should be placed close to (but not necessarily on) your desk. You should have two other bins, one for magazines and journals, and one for other non-priority mail such as lecture brochures.

Finally, eliminate your "time traps." For at least one week, keep track of your time in a notebook. Record your daily events (such as 7:00–7:30 a.m., attend staff meeting; 7:30–8:30 a.m., hospital rounds). If you detect any time traps, eliminate them. Also, reorganize your schedule to take advantage of your most efficient times. For instance, if you know you are most productive between 1 p.m. and 4 p.m., avoid scheduling afternoon meetings.

Maximizing your time by staying organized is not an isolated effort. It requires continuous commitment from you and your staff. By improving your working conditions and habits, you will enhance your productive ability and perhaps even gain some well-earned personal time.

David Woods

Technology to enhance your practice

Where does the Internet fit in between your office, your patients, and your own continuing medical education?

A good rule of thumb is to always choose technology that helps your patients in some way. With that in mind, start with the Online Software Consultant (www.health-infosys-dir.com/yp_hc.asp), a convenient resource featuring detailed descriptions of technology vendors and websites listed by healthcare category.

WebMD (www.webmd.com) offers comprehensive and integrated solutions for your practice. Their mission is to provide products and services that help "promote efficiency and reduce costs" by facilitating communication amongst all healthcare participants. WebMD Intergy, one of their practice management systems, enables you to quickly access all patient information from a central location for easier appointment scheduling, accounting, and reporting. Another system, The Medical Manager, includes document and image management as well as wireless and Internet connectivity. WebMD can also help you securely interact with your own practice management systems from handheld devices or from your home computer. Such flexibility enables you to move forward at your own pace toward an almost entirely paperless office, significantly reducing errors while improving patient care.

If you're looking for customized medical information, WebMD Health is the leading consumer-focused healthcare information website. You and your patients can access health news, online support communities, and interactive health management tools, as well as participate in real-time discussions with medical experts. There's also Medscape's Patient Education Center, which has over 575 000 registered physicians and 1.6 million healthcare professionals worldwide whose mission is to provide "objective, credible, and relevant" clinical information and educational tools. The site is continually updated with coverage of medical conferences, access to over 100 medical journals, and specialty-specific daily medical news. Everything can be printed for reading offline.

One of the simplest and most effective tools for your patients is your own website. A website is inexpensive and can provide office hours, directions, and background information about you and your staff. It can also provide answers to your most commonly asked questions and even include links to some of the information-based websites mentioned above. By providing this key information online, you'll help market your practice and reduce unnecessary calls to your office.

Jonathan Coopersmith

Healthscapes: how physical surroundings influence perceptions of quality

As healthcare becomes more competitive and the desire to measure and achieve quality becomes more urgent, it seems odd that a factor as influential as the so-called healthscape remains the object of so little attention.

Hospital and doctors' waiting rooms are still all too often drab and forbidding places stocked with ancient periodicals, wilting plants, tacky furniture, and a generally unwelcoming layout. Not that anyone wants to be in either of those places, but if they are, then the experience should surely be made as "user-friendly" as possible.

What that means is paying attention to such ambient conditions as temperature, air quality, noise, music, odor, colors, lighting, and texture; space and function factors such as crowding, layout, equipment, and furnishings; and signs and symbols such as "wayfinding," personal artifacts, and decor.

At the highest level of abstraction, humans have sought positive identification with their physical surroundings since cave dwellers painted their walls in prehistoric times. In modern healthcare, if patients receive treatment in a run-down facility, they are likely to demean not only the facility but the treatment as well. Patients who are "dissatisfied" with a facility are more likely to switch to another.

Healthscapes will be of paramount concern to marketers because of health-care's low price differential, inseparability of service and place – and increasing competition.

Organized and tidy environments are more likely to lead to satisfaction with a healthcare facility than disorganized ones. A basic human instinct is to want to feel safe in a given environment. Surroundings must be kept clean, organized, pleasant smelling, and comfortable, without going overboard with plush sur-roundings. All areas of health facilities must be accessible to as much natural light as possible. Noise and temperature levels should be monitored and maintained.

If a patient is more satisfied with the healthscape of a healthcare facility, then he or she is more likely to be satisfied with the complete service encounter. Most important, proper healthscapes can have a positive impact upon the actual healing processes of patients.

David Woods

Hiring? Use this checklist

If you are hiring a new doctor for your practice, settle these fundamental issues before you make an offer or draft an employment agreement.

Total compensation

Compensation only starts with salary. Estimate the costs of expected benefits, including:

- malpractice insurance
- hospital staff dues
- licensing fees
- professional society dues
- beeper
- continuing medical education.

Benefits that may make your offer more attractive than your competitors' offers include:

- board examination fees
- automobile allowance
- cellular phone
- moving expenses.

Total the costs of all benefits you intend to offer before you promise a particular salary and bonus.

Termination

Unexpected, occasionally hostile, practice "break-ups" do happen. Carefully draft appropriate termination language, including:

- "no cause" termination (with 30, 60, or 90 days' notice)
- "for cause" termination for immediate dismissal upon the occurrence of a serious event, such as loss of medical license
- competition covenants – a departing associate could take some of your business away.

Protect your practice

A restrictive covenant prohibits your associate from practicing within a certain distance from your practice for a certain period after termination.

A non-solicitation covenant prohibits your employee from soliciting your patients, office staff, referring physicians, or practice contacts.

Ownership arrangements

If you may ultimately offer your new doctor "partnership," include the terms of the ownership arrangement ("buy-in") in the employment agreement. You may prevent problems, such as an associate refusing to compensate you for the value of your practice, when it is time for the associate to buy into your practice.

Expectations and boundaries

Use your employment agreement to:

- establish evaluation criteria, including frequency of evaluation
- prevent non-approved "moonlighting" for another entity
- affirm that, until such time as he or she becomes a co-owner, your associate has no ownership interest in your practice and thus is not entitled to: accounts receivable, patient lists, referring physician lists, patient records.

Use these issues as a loose framework.

Always have an adviser, who is familiar with drafting new doctor employment and co-ownership arrangements, to help you plan and draft your employment agreements.

How to handle complaints

Many of us avoid handling complaints because we don't feel skilled at responding to them. We know how we like to be treated when we have a complaint, but when the complaint is about us or our organization, apprehension sets in. As a result, we often act defensively and make non-helpful statements such as "Well, you are the only person who has ever complained about this," or "No one in this office would ever say such a thing."

Each time you have a complaint, observe how it is handled and think about whether the positives and negatives are transferable to your practice or organization. An effective staff exercise is to ask employees about any recent complaints they had – why they did or didn't voice them and how they were resolved. Make a list of the positive and negative ways their complaints were handled and ask for suggestions about better complaint-handling in your practice.

When a patient voices a complaint, create a mindset for yourself that *a complaint is a good thing*. Although you may not like what you hear, you should want to hear it. Many doctors think the patient is cured, when he or she has merely quit in disgust. Indeed, many patients would rather choose another doctor than complain. Make it easy for patients to communicate how they feel. Patient satisfaction surveys tell patients that you want to hear about ways to improve your care and service. A survey can be as simple as three questions:

- What do you like best about our practice?
- What do you like least?
- What could we provide for you that we are not offering now?

When you receive a complaint, use these strategies:

- Don't mirror the patient's tone of voice if he or she is angry or upset. Mirroring or responding with annoyance, impatience, or anger only escalates conflict.
- If the complaint is unreasonable, say nothing and permit the person's words to land and to echo back.
- Take advantage of the complainer's right to be right by finding something that they are right about and reinforcing it. "You're right, Mrs Smith. The office does get hectic in the afternoons."
- When you have done something that justifies a complaint, you may be inclined to say "I'm sorry" as a way to get past the conflict. An example might be if you were late arriving one morning, resulting in a long wait for your patient. "I'm sorry," offered too quickly and without feeling, can send the message "OK, I've done my part – if you're still upset, it's your problem. I've apologized." An alternative to "I'm sorry" is "Please forgive me." This statement sends a message that returns control to the patient. Think about why "Please forgive me" might be an uncomfortable statement for you. It may be that you have been taught that it is critically important that your decisions are the correct ones. Your image as a competent professional depends on this. Don't let your

need to be right, to have all the answers, prevent you from showing empathy and thus push people away.
- Assurance of an ongoing relationship is the technique that differentiates the novice from the skilled complaint handler. Statements such as "I'll be on duty until 11 p.m. – ask for me if there is anything else I can do for you" or "Please tell me if this situation ever occurs again" let the patient know that it's okay to complain and that you want the relationship to continue.

When patients complain, they want four things: someone to listen, someone to care, someone to take action, and someone to assure them of an ongoing relationship. Respond to these wants by doing the following:

- *Listen*. Listen without interruption: "Tell me why you feel that way;" "Tell me the whole story;" "That must have been very difficult for you".
- *Action*. Be clear about what each of you will do when the conversation ends. What, specifically, have you promised to do? Who will call whom? When?
- *Assure*. Ice the cake with a statement such as "I'm sorry you had to wait. You are one of my favorite patients and I want your visits here to be as convenient and pleasant as possible. Thank you for your understanding about the scheduling problem that occurred today. We'll make sure that your next appointment is the first appointment of the afternoon and we'll do our best to see you right on time."

Recognize that a complaint has two messages. One is the issue that the patient seems to be dissatisfied about. The second message is "I want this relationship to continue. Help straighten this out for me." Maintain and strengthen your relationship by seeing that both messages are acknowledged!

Susan Keane Baker

How to respond to an angry complaint

An angry complaint can ruin your day. You have to spend extra time dealing with the patient. Extra time spent listening to your staff's side of the story. Extra time spent thinking about the situation and how you could have responded differently. Here are some steps for handling angry complaints so that they don't consume more time and energy than is necessary:

- Move the patient to a quiet area of the practice. In a low, calm tone of voice, say to the patient, "Let's step over here to talk. That way, we won't be interrupted." The angry patient with an audience will be less likely to accept your point of view, even if he comes to understand your position. And if during the course of that conversation you make a concession, you may be creating expectations for other patients that if they become loud and boisterous you'll do the same for them.
- Let the patient speak his mind without interruption. Otherwise, you may fix the problem, but not fix the relationship. You may be encouraging the patient to embellish and repeat his story to others, since he hasn't been heard by you.
- Avoid rationalizing. There are usually a few oft-repeated rationalizations that come immediately to mind when a patient has a complaint: "It's the insurance companies;" "It's the way we've always done it." Put yourself in the patient's shoes for just a moment and consider whether your rationalization is an explanation or an excuse.
- Respectfully use the patient's name in your reply. When a person is very angry, using his or her name in a respectful way can ease the situation. Using the person's name in a condescending way fuels anger.
- Demonstrate your understanding. If sincere, use the "feel, felt, found" technique. For example, "I understand how you feel. I've felt that way too when I've received a bill that didn't seem to make any sense. What I've found is that writing down my questions for the billing people helps us both understand where the misunderstandings are and resolve the problem without anyone's feelings being hurt."
- Resist the urge to escalate the situation. As Donald Snook, a former hospital CEO with many years of conflict resolution experience, says, "Escalation is the easiest thing to do, but it's no fun." Keep your own frustrations, temptation to blame others, and pride in check. Keep one goal in mind: to resolve the issue in a way that preserves your relationship with your patient. Using these strategies will help you resolve conflict more positively, and give you peace of mind that you handled the situation in a professional, dignified manner. And that's what frees up your mind and your time for more positive, productive activities.

Susan Keane Baker

How to improve your sign language

Signs that patients see while visiting your practice send messages. Some messages are those you intended when you ordered the sign or allowed your staff to post it. Others signal things you might not have considered. Take a fresh look at all the postings in your practice and ask yourself, "If I were a new patient, how would I feel when reading this?"

- *Waiting Room.* This sign says "You can expect to wait." Substitute "Reception" to indicate that this is where patients will be greeted warmly.
- *We try to see patients in order of appointment, not arrival.* This sign can ease some tensions in your reception area, as patients who arrive early sit fuming while later but "appointment on time" arrivals are ushered straight in.
- *The worst day at the beach is better than the greatest day at work.* These signs may be humorous, and some employees might say motivational, but they belong in areas of your practice that are out of patients' view.
- *Payment is expected at the time of service unless other arrangements have been made.* Patients who have no intention of paying the bill that day will assume that if other arrangements have ever been made, they can be made for them too. Patients who do pay at the time of service may wonder whether your "preferred" patients get to make other arrangements. Change this sign to "Payment is expected at the time of service." Period. The "unless other arrangements" part goes without saying. Those who want or need the other arrangements will let you know.
- *Bravery not allowed in this office.* Some patients like this sign, feeling that it's all right to be nervous and that you have a sense of humor, too. Others may feel that you're sending a message that pain is about to be inflicted.
- *Will the following patients kindly see the office manager regarding unpaid accounts.* Get rid of this one. We're talking breach of confidentiality here.
- *We participate in the following health plans: ABC, Yourchoice, HIJ, Backs R Us.* Patients like the reassurance that you are still accepting their insurance. Also, they may be able to recall which plans you accept when they next have to select a health plan at work.
- *Our Team: physician partners, nurse, practice manager, receptionist.* Signs in the reception area identifying staff are well received by patients. If your staff protests against name tags, signs like these give patients a chance to connect on a more personal level. It's easier to ask questions of someone if you know his or her name.
- *Please leave your urine specimen on the shelf next to the sink.* Signs like this help ease "anxiety of the uninitiated." Instead of paying attention to the nurse's instructions about where to leave the specimen, the new patient may be thinking "Where is the bathroom?" "Why did I use the bathroom before I

left work?'' ''Will anyone knock on the door while I'm in there?'' ''Can the people in the reception area hear me?'' A sign that reminds the patient of what to do next helps him or her do the right thing.

* *Please tell us if there has been any change in your medical condition since your last visit.* A sign like this in the examination room, not the reception area, can be a risk-management safety net for the doctor. It tells patients that you are concerned about what happened to them between visits.

Of course, too many signs plastered about can give the appearance of a poorly organized practice. When considering signs, think about the questions patients frequently ask. Think about whether the sign is there for your benefit or theirs. Test possible signs on a few patients. People love to give their opinion – take advantage of this to improve the service of your practice.

Susan Keane Baker

A complete, updated and signed history is vital before treatment begins

In many alleged misdiagnoses of breast cancer, the history the patient gives to you becomes very important.

In a recent US case, it was admitted that there was a thickening in the upper, outer quadrant of the breast in a 44-year-old woman; a mammogram had been ordered, which reported the study was essentially consistent with fibrocystic disease. The mammographer did suggest clinical correlation and further follow-up testing in six months. The family doctor reasoned that, since the patient had a benign history, he could reassure her. What he said was, "This is going to be fine, there doesn't seem to be a problem here; why don't you just follow up in six months?"

The patient did not follow up in six months and, in fact, didn't see a healthcare provider for 14 months. When she did, she was found to have carcinoma of the breast, which had metastasized to the lymph nodes. At the same time, it was determined that she did indeed have a family history of breast cancer, a fact the family doctor denied knowledge of when she sued him for misdiagnosis. His office history form had been partly completed, but the patient's signature had not been appended to it. Why didn't the complete history form get filled out? Why didn't the patient follow up? Why is the doctor concerned about this lawsuit?

There were two lapses of communication. First, the history form was made to seem as if it were a formality. The patient was asked to fill out the form while waiting in the reception area during her first visit years ago. She did so, and at that time there was no family history of breast cancer. But in the interim, her grandmother had died of breast cancer and her maternal aunt was being treated for the disease.

Why didn't the patient make the physician aware of this? Why did she not update her history? Some patients tend not to focus on the importance of their family history. Others are simply in denial that a health problem affecting other family members could happen to them. Law books and defense lawyers' filing cabinets are filled with documents about patients who have denied their symptoms, are diagnosed late, and then complain that they had informed their physicians time and time again of their symptoms.

In reality, it simply didn't happen, and now, in the face of this devastating disease, they are unwilling to accept the responsibility.

The physician should let patients know, both on the history form and during discussions with them, how important it is to give an accurate history and to update it regularly. In fact, at the beginning of the history form there should be a sentence reading: "The following information is very important to us in taking care of your health. Please take the time to completely and accurately fill out all of this information. Please also make sure you update this information as changes occur." At the end of the form have a line where the patient signs with the statement: "The above information is true and correct to the best of my belief." This simply underscores how important the process is.

Second, when reassuring a patient, take great care to balance your reassurance with the need to follow up with scheduled appointments since the situation still needs to be carefully monitored. Most patients do not want to hear even potential bad news. So when good news is given, patients will often let it completely absorb them. Letting them know, when appropriate, how imperative follow-up is balances the conversation out.

In this case, clear communication that follow-up in six months was not an option but part of the treatment plan was critical. An appointment could have been set up on that day. Further, many physicians have a recall system in circumstances such as this, whereby a phone call would be made or a postcard would go out if the visit was not kept. Again, a few words in these situations could have made a big difference and, as always, documentation of them is also vital.

James Saxton

Making your reception area more welcoming

The environment of your reception area creates clues for people about what they should realistically expect from the care and service in your practice. Too elaborate an area may send a message that care will be expensive, while an overcrowded room full of grouchy-looking people signals a long wait and a rushed physician.

Some practices take advantage of the reception experience by providing relevant health and practice information; by staffing the area with a gracious person who is truly interested in helping patients feel comfortable; and by using scheduling protocols that keep waits to 15 minutes or less. Here are some additional techniques:

- Keep your practice brochures in your reception area. It's an easy way for people to refresh their recollections about how your practice works.
- Make available the latest patient satisfaction survey comments. Seeing that you care about the comments will encourage more people to complete the survey, and you will have a steady stream of patient compliments to entertain guests in your reception area. If there is a coffee table in your reception area, have a piece of glass cut to fit on top and create an exhibit area for information you would like your patients to read.
- Provide the names of all members of the practice, with their titles and functions, and perhaps their photos, too. It's easier for people to approach a staff member when they can recall the person's name. It also sends a message that every person on staff is a respected member of the team.
- Have a selection of reading material that reflects the interests of your patients. Avoid creating a perception that "it's all about me" by having magazines that reflect your – rather than your patients' – interests.
- Listen when people talk about their impressions and experiences. One woman mentioned to a pediatrician that she was upset when her well children were exposed to sick children in the reception area. He agreed, and turned a supply room into a sick-child area, where waiting children are seen faster. Being seen faster is the incentive for parents of sick children to take them to that area rather than keeping them in the well-child space.
- The best feature of any reception area is immediate acknowledgement of people as they arrive. A warm welcome creates a positive expectation about the care and service that will follow and builds trust and rapport. The most savvy physicians make it an essential part of their practice.

Susan Keane Baker

Minimizing risk

Communication and documentation at the root of growing legal risks

The revolution in healthcare has brought with it a tangled array of legal risks for physicians that far transcend the traditional one doctor, one patient, one episode suit for real or imagined negligence. Among the new risks are contract and credentialing issues involving prospective physician members of a group, coverage and utilization decisions, and cost constraints, including devolution of care to mid-level professionals.

Physicians can minimize legal risk by creating a culture of quality, by aggressively confronting patient anger and mitigating it to stave off litigation after a potential compensable event, and by dissuading plaintiffs' attorneys from taking the case by having watertight contracts and patient records.

With a growing number of medical malpractice suits now originating in physicians' offices, administrative risk in that setting is increasing. And a fast-growing area of litigation is diagnosis-related because of the impact of gate-keeping for large patient groups for which attempts to determine what can or should be done are affected by cost constraints on procedures and tests. The solution is to standardize protocols and to delegate to nurse practitioners and physician assistants, although that in itself may incur risk if these people are improperly credentialed or inadequately supervised. It is not a lack of technical skill that leads to the three top allegations in a suit involving a practice setting – failure to diagnose, failure to treat, and medication errors – but inadequate follow-through and tracking. Time constraints on primary care physicians particularly may lead to inadequate assessments, skimpy or inaccurate documentation and communication, poor follow-up (inclusive of no-shows), and missed test results because there is no coordination or because they go unread.

It is up to the physician to put in place standards of judgment and care, office systems that ensure proper continuity (including after-hours coverage), to look closely at credentials of staff, and to develop patient satisfaction reports.

In the new world of healthcare, physicians need to pick their way carefully through a minefield of legal risks, the most potentially explosive of which are contracts, credentials, delegation, utilization, multiple providers dealing with groups of patients in a continuum of care – and inadequate communication and documentation.

David Woods

Clean up your documentation: use SOAP

One needs to understand what lawyers are doing with documentation. Although it used to be that medical charts were merely numbered as exhibits in courtrooms and at times shown to the jury, now particular records that are helpful to either side are blown up $3' \times 5'$ (at least) and put on posterboard. This just drives home the importance of good documentation, which will become more important as laws concerning fraud and abuse and audits become more prevalent. Further, professional liability documentation can discourage a plaintiff from pursuing a claim, discourage a plaintiff's lawyer from taking on a case, or discourage a highly regarded expert from supporting such an action.

Documentation of your plan and the basis for your actions is now more important than ever. How else can one determine several years down the road why a certain course of treatment was being followed? Simply throwing up your hands, indicating "it wasn't my decision" or "my hands were tied," will not work.

Although an enormous amount of material has been written about documentation, at times it is good to get back to the basics. The SOAP has always been one of the cornerstones for organizing good documentation – **S**etting forth your subjective analysis of what you are seeing, hearing, and feeling, followed by your **O**bjective findings, your **A**ssessment, and then, most important, your **P**lan, and doing so routinely goes a long way to providing the baseline protection you need.

"Routinely" is the action word that makes this all work. One must be disciplined to use every letter and to describe each part of the SOAP formula. Inconsistency is the downfall of good documentation.

Documentation has always been important. However, in the environment in which physicians find themselves practicing today, it has taken on new importance. No longer is it something that just the "lawyers" want. It is essential for physicians to understand that failing to document appropriately can expose one not only to a greater likelihood of professional negligence claims but to challenges in a reimbursement context or even a licensing issue. A starting point: at random, pull three of your charts and see if you have really documented the good care you have provided. If not, get your systems in place.

James Saxton

Telephone advice should be documented

As doctors see ever more patients and do so with fewer resources, there is a trend toward handling more complaints, questions, and concerns by telephone.

Questions about medications, physical therapy, pre- and postoperative instructions always occur. However, there will also be more calls of a clinical nature. A patient calls the primary care physician wondering if a condition is serious enough to warrant an emergency department visit. A parent calls the pediatrician to determine whether a visit to the pediatrician's office is needed that afternoon or whether the symptoms are just a normal progression of the child's disease. Important clinical decision making is occurring over the phone more and more often. And when there is a legal problem, this practice is scrutinized and often ascribed to economic motivation – an aggravating factor to any jury.

Often, people on the front line, the medical receptionist for example, are handling these calls. They do so in the best way they can, but we must remember that they need the tools to do so effectively. They need to know when to refer the call to a nurse or a physician. They need to have some training or to be asking – or answering –within a framework of protocol or policy. The receptionist may not be equipped to ask the right questions to discern whether the patient needs a visit to the emergency department, a follow-up appointment with the doctor's office, or an emergency visit to the doctor's office.

When a nurse, nurse practitioner, or the doctor handles calls, enough time has to be spent to determine whether or not an immediate referral is necessary. The classic example is a telephone call to the primary care "gatekeeper's" home via their service at night. The patient has symptoms that he or she feels might be a myocardial infarction. The doctor has to act prudently as a so-called gatekeeper in determining whether an emergency department visit is called for in the circumstances or whether a visit to the physician's office the next day will suffice. Certainly, in these circumstances, the way the information is communicated back and forth is critical. Many suggest that if a non-physician is handling this call, certain methods or protocols should be developed so that precise questions are asked. Further, if someone goes through a plethora of questions, responses should be recorded and documented; in the event of litigation, having that call documented is critical.

James Saxton

The telephone: instrument of the devil or practice enhancer?

Every telephone call to your practice is a moment of truth for the caller. For some, it is the first moment and therefore critically important to the impression they will form about you and how satisfied they expect to be with your medical care. Here are some ways to enhance your practice by the care you give on the telephone:

- Use a consistent opening. Patients are comforted that they have reached the right place when they hear the same message. Get your staff together and decide how the telephone should be answered. Then post the script until it becomes a habit. "Thank you for calling Norwood Medical Group, this is Mary," or "Thank you for calling Norwood Medical Group, how may I help you?" are two options.
- Listen carefully for the caller's name. Most of us listen for what the call is about, forgetting that our relationship with the caller comes first. It is far more effective to get the caller's name at the outset.
- Use the caller's name at least once during the conversation.
- Put a positive spin on your standard responses. Instead of just giving directions, add a patient-pleasing comment such as "We're in a lovely white Victorian house across from Riverview Park."
- Try to use "for you" at least once during the conversation, for example: "I'll be happy to give Dr Thompson the message for you. We'll call the prescription in for you this afternoon." This takes a second, but subtly reminds the patient that you are taking care of him or her.
- Try to incorporate a "statement of caring" into the discussion. When you really listen, you pick up on items that may not be relevant to the call but certainly are relevant to the patients and your relationship with them. For example: "This is John Smith. I'm calling to cancel my appointment because my son's team has made the play-offs and he has a game the same time as my visit with you." You can reschedule the appointment, addressing the caller's needs. But if you add "Have a great time at the game, I hope they win," you've made the call special.
- Be clear about who will do what next. "Let me recap what we've discussed. You're going to call Dr Jones and ask her to send us your medical records. As soon as we receive them I'll call you to set up an appointment. If you don't hear from me within three weeks, please call me to check on what's happening."
- At the end of every call, no matter how brief, ask: "Is there anything else I can do for you today?" There won't be anything else 99% of the time, but 100% of callers will hang up feeling very well taken care of.

Susan Keane Baker

Ten tips for effective informed consent discussions

Giving a patient an "informed consent" paper to sign after a procedure, or giving a form to sign that is too technical for the patient to understand, provides you little protection in the event of a suit alleging lack of the patient's prior informed consent. You are aware that performing a procedure without obtaining the patient's informed consent is considered assault and/or battery. The informed consent discussion is vital to managing the patient's expectations and your malpractice risk. Here are some tips for making the discussion more valuable for you and your patient:

1 Ask your patient what he or she knows about the procedure before you describe it. For example, asking "Have any of your family members or friends ever had this procedure? What did they tell you about it?" gives the patient an opportunity to express knowledge without worrying about appearing uninformed. Finding out what the patient knows gives you an opportunity to discern expectations, misconceptions, and probable questions.

2 After describing the nature and scope of the procedure, including the proposed benefits and possible risks, outline your patient's alternatives. Be sure that one option is doing nothing.

3 If your patient declines treatment, be conscientious about enumerating the risks of not undergoing the procedure. Don't leave yourself open to claims of failure to diagnose or delay diagnosis claims because you didn't impress the patient enough or failed to check that the patient followed through. Documenting the refusal is as important as documenting the consent.

4 If you or your professional association have prepared written materials about the procedure you are proposing, use the materials as a guide for your discussion. Check off the most pertinent points before giving the materials to your patient.

5 After discussing the nature of the procedure, the risks, benefits, and alternatives, ask your patient "Now that we've discussed your alternatives, what would you like me to do?" The patient who can't respond or says something like "Whatever you think best, doctor" is not adequately prepared to give an informed consent.

6 Instead of asking "Do you have any questions?" ask "What questions do you have?" or "What questions can I answer for you?"

7 During the consent discussion, the patient may be thinking that a second opinion may be necessary but is afraid of hurting your feelings by broaching the subject. You will appear confident and compassionate by introducing the topic yourself. "If you would like to get a second opinion before authorizing

this procedure, I will be happy to send a copy of your chart, X-rays, or test results to another physician."

8   If your patient has unrealistic expectations, you can empathize while setting the record straight. "I wish that you would be 100% pain-free after the operation, but most patients experience pain for at least a few weeks afterwards."

9   If your patient speaks another language, be very careful about whom you use as a translator. If you use a family member or staff member with limited medical training, you run the risk that the person may interpret incorrectly.

10   When your patient makes a decision to proceed, reinforce the wisdom or courage of the decision. "I know that this is not an easy decision, but this is certainly what I would do if I were you." Be careful that your reinforcement is not a guarantee or a statement that will create unrealistic expectations. Don't say "I know this is tough, but after the surgery you'll feel like a new person."

The consent discussion is one of the most important interactions you ever have with your patient. Don't delegate the discussion to someone else. Don't become so annoyed by bureaucratic red tape that you avoid the process altogether. An informed patient is a more compliant patient. A more compliant patient is more likely to have a better outcome. A patient with a good outcome is more likely to be satisfied.

Susan Keane Baker

Top ten issues in medical malpractice

While physicians must be educated about some new issues when practicing in today's environment, most malpractice trials still concern many of the old tried and true medical legal problems.

1 *Communications issues* would be top. Not only issues involving communication between physician and patient, but physicians with other treating or consulting physicians, physicians with other healthcare providers, physicians with office staff or hospital staff, and between patient and the physician office staff, to name a few. Communication issues may also lead to allegations of failure to follow up or failure to diagnose in a timely manner.
2 *Documentation*, including the issues of legibility, confidentiality, and technology, e.g. faxing of medical records, use of e-mail, and computerized medical records.
3 *Confidentiality* regarding the medical record, especially when pertaining to HIV, psychiatric diagnoses, and any drug or alcohol problems that are documented in a patient's chart; also, confidentiality in the physician office setting. An example would be notification of test results in a non-confidential manner.
4 *Telephone issues*. Again, the issue of confidentiality, prescribing medications on the phone, and making diagnoses on the phone would be areas of concern. Another would be the use of cellular phones and thus the possibility of being overheard.
5 *Telemedicine*. From a liability perspective, telemedicine is a growing field. The issues include licensure; malpractice policy; credentialing of the physician involved; informed consent; and ownership of records – written, audio, or video.
6 *Informed consent* is also an issue that seems to hover whenever a malpractice suit is initiated. Elements of adequate informed consent include documentation about the nature of the illness, recommended treatment, purpose of the treatment, likelihood of success, inherent risks, and the consequences of no treatment.
7 *Modification* of biomedical equipment and off-label use.
8 *Regulations* concerning the duty to report by a physician regarding elder abuse, spousal abuse, child abuse, reporting certain infectious diseases, and reporting certain medical conditions.
9 *Management issues*, which may include but not be limited to advertising, utilization review, contracts, benefit administration and denials, accreditation compliance, physician credentialing, clinical guidelines and protocols, and fraud and abuse regulations.
10 *Ethics*. ''Do not resuscitate,'' medication errors, genetic testing, reuse of single-use products, and the emotional issue of assisted suicide.

Robert Pendrak MD

You've been called as an expert witness: now what?

Whether it is for plaintiff or defendant healthcare provider, or as an expert in a personal injury case, being an expert witness is a serious task and one in which either party will rely heavily on your guidance and, ultimately, your testimony.

If you are asked to be an expert, count on being asked to review not only the medical records but also copies of deposition transcripts, perhaps opposing expert reports, pleadings in the lawsuit, statements or answers to what are referred to as interrogatories (which are merely questions one side poses to the other in written form), and perhaps literature that has been submitted on behalf of the opposing party.

The expert must be willing to take the time to provide the party who has requested his or her guidance with some help and instruction on framing the issues and, potentially, preparing for cross-examination of the opposing expert. You may be asked to do a literature search in an effort not only to support your conclusions but to help discredit the opponent's conclusions.

You must be prepared to be called to testify at trial. Although experts are sometimes seen only on videotape, more often than not they are asked to attend trial. Be prepared to subject yourself not just to direct examination by the party calling you, but to cross-examination by the opposing counsel. Many experts say that the time during which they are cross-examined is extremely stressful and similar to having to submit to a specialty examination. You will need to be prepared for direct examination so your testimony should be smooth, under-standable, and communicated in such a way that a jury understands it. You need to understand the opposing party's themes and theories so that questions are not in a vacuum. You should be prepared for the types of questions to which the participating lawyers normally resort.

As with any important task, preparation is the key.

James Saxton

Terminating the physician–patient relationship

Physicians who are sued for malpractice are often heard to say, "I knew the person was bad news. I kept thinking he or she would just go away, or that I could change things. I didn't terminate the relationship because I just didn't want to be mean."

Physicians would be well advised to document evidence of patient dissatisfaction. This evidence might include a pattern of failure to follow through with agreed-upon treatment recommendations, written or oral complaints to you or your staff, or chronic failure to keep appointments. Seeing a pattern of dissatisfaction over time may signal to you that the patient might do better in the care of another physician.

If you decide to terminate your relationship with a patient, check with your liability carriers to see if they have a protocol to be followed and a letter to be sent. A commonly found protocol for terminating a patient relationship is as follows:

1   Send a certified letter, return receipt requested. Some attorneys suggest using restricted delivery, meaning that the letter is signed for by the addressee only.
2   Keep a copy of the letter and attach it to the patient's medical record.
3   Give no reason or a general reason for the termination.
4   Offer routine medical care for the first 15 days from the date of the letter.
5   Offer emergency care for the second 15 days from the date of the letter.
6   Offer to send copies of the patient's medical records to a new physician, whether or not the patient owes you a balance. Don't specifically name other physicians for the patient to consider. Instead, provide the contact information for the medical society's physician referral program.
7   State that the relationship will be terminated 30 days from the date of the letter.
8   Note any subsequent communication you have with the patient.

As in other relationships, the patient may be reluctant to let go. Be sure that your partners and support staff are aware that the relationship has been terminated, so that the patient doesn't re-establish the relationship by obtaining a prescription refill from someone on call.

Physicians who have terminated relations with patients report that some will ask for another chance. What should you do when you've finally taken the difficult step of terminating the relationship and your patient contacts you, begging to return? If you are going to go to the trouble of terminating the relationship, don't reinstate the patient if you have even the slightest reservation about doing so.

Susan Keane Baker

Quiz

Are you a good communicator?

Technology has not changed the most crucial aspects of a physician's work – interacting with patients. Here is a quiz to help you gauge your own communication skills.

Circle the one best answer to each question. Answer honestly with your first instinct rather than trying for the "right" answer. Leave the score line blank until you've completed the quiz and read the scoring instructions at the end.

1   When I see the words "doctor–patient communication," I first think of:
    (a)   spoken language exchanged during an encounter
    (b)   everything that's said, as well as subtle cues, body language, and listening skills
    (c)   all of the above, plus attributes of empathy, concern, and touch.

2   My own postgraduate training in communication skills included:
    (a)   videotaped interviews with model patients
    (b)   classroom material and lectures
    (c)   none of the above.

3   In general, my philosophy about getting along with patients is:
    (a)   some patients will like me, others won't. Those who don't will eventually find another physician
    (b)   I make a good-faith effort to establish a working relationship with every new patient, but sometimes it just doesn't work out
    (c)   I work hard to earn the trust of every new patient, even those who are "difficult." I rarely fail to make a connection, but it doesn't always happen right away.

4   If I were to attend a continuing medical education retreat, the speaker or doctor–patient communication would find me:
    (a)   listening attentively in the front half of the room
    (b)   in the room, but probably thinking about something else or refilling my coffee cup
    (c)   absent, probably on the golf course.

5   When a patient in the exam room takes out a handwritten list of questions to ask me, I typically respond by:
    (a)   groaning inwardly
    (b)   addressing the list hurriedly, aware that I'm falling behind in my schedule
    (c)   recognizing the list as a helpful tool, and scheduling follow-up time.

6   When a visit with a patient has gone badly, I usually:
    (a)   find out about it later, in an angry letter or telephone complaint
    (b)   know it by the end of the interview, but reassure myself that I can't please everyone

(c) realize it right away, and ask the patient to help me understand expectations and where breakdown occurred.

7 When I am faced with a puzzling diagnosis or an unusual constellation of symptoms, my next step is usually to:
(a) refer to a consultant
(b) repeat my physical exam and order more tests
(c) review the patient's history, inviting the patient to brainstorm.

8 Were a patient to make a formal complaint about my care, I would:
(a) respond to the patient promptly, and resolve the concerns as best I could
(b) forward the complaint to a staff member to handle
(c) call my malpractice carrier.

9 Compared with colleagues who practice in the same area as I do, I have been involved in malpractice actions:
(a) more than my peers
(b) about the same as my peers
(c) less than my peers.

SCORING: All odd numbered questions score 0 for an A answer, 1 for B, 2 for C. Even numbered questions score the reverse: 2 for A, 1 for B, 0 for C. Enter each score above, then subtotal your score to the nine questions. Enter 2 points here if you read the text preceding the quiz, 0 if not. TOTAL:

How do you compare?

16–20. You already know how important good communication with your patients is. Your practice is probably thriving.

11–15. Don't be discouraged. You have made a good-faith effort to develop effective communication skills, but perhaps you need to work on some areas.

10 or lower. You are faced with a challenge – and an opportunity. It might be time to devote your next continuing medical education class to updating your skills. The art of communication, as intangible as it may seem, is measurable and teachable.

Albert Mehl MD

Patient questionnaire

Ask your receptionist to distribute copies of the following survey questionnaire as patients enter your office and collect them as they leave. Put a box in the office in which patients can leave completed questionnaires. If necessary, give patients self-addressed, stamped envelopes to mail in forms they complete at home.

Ensuring and proving patient satisfaction is too important to your medical practice to leave to chance. If you need professional help to survey your patients, analyze the results, and plan the changes, get it.

How would you rate the following, on a scale of 1 (poor) to 10 (excellent)?

Receptionist's:
courtesy: ☐
knowledge: ☐
helpfulness: ☐

Doctor's:
patience: ☐
interest in your problem: ☐
amount of time spent with you: ☐
explanation: ☐
treatment: ☐

Clinical staff's:
knowledge: ☐
helpfulness: ☐

Facility's:
appearance: ☐
comfort: ☐
cleanliness: ☐
other features: ☐
reception area: ☐
waiting room: ☐
examination room's privacy: ☐

General quality of medical care you received: ☐

How did you get to our office?

How many miles did you travel?

Parking availability (circle one):
Excellent   Good   Fair   Poor

Parking security (circle one):
Excellent   Good   Fair   Poor

How many days did you wait for your appointment?

How long after your scheduled appointment time did you wait before seeing the doctor?

Are you satisfied with our office hours?

Please tell us what you would change and how you would change it:

Which of the following influenced your decision to use our office?
Referred by: another patient; a doctor; a family member; physician referral service

Index